FREE YOURSELF FROM THE GRIP OF ALCOHOL ADDICTION

10 SIMPLE STEPS TO ACHIEVE SOBRIETY, ENHANCE MENTAL AND PHYSICAL WELL-BEING, STRENGTHEN RELATIONSHIPS, AND OVERCOME SELF-DOUBT

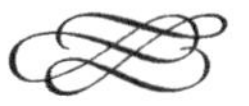

YVONNE L.M. CROSS

CONTENTS

INTRODUCTION

I want to say that I was always a drinker. I started drinking when I was just eight years old. I wasn't always drunk, but I always drank more when something tragic happened in my life, but it would calm down after a period of time. I started drinking more heavily, and my addiction spiraled out of control on the day my fiance, the love of my life, was taken off of life support. After 10 days in an induced coma and four more months in the hospital with pancreatitis, he had a heart attack because his body couldn't take anymore. After that day, I felt like life would never be okay again, and I plummeted.

Once again, I was parked in a seat at the bar, cradling a shot in one hand and a cold beer in the other. Only this time, I was not sitting with my fiancé; I was alone and in tears. I had just made that heartbreaking decision to permit the doctor to remove my love from life support, allowing him to be freed from the pain and suffering caused by his pancreatitis.

It was an especially hard decision to make, knowing that he also struggled with a drinking problem, just like me.

What am I going to do now? Our love, real estate business, and my world had just been turned upside down.

"I know ..." my brain began to offer, the same as with every other tragedy in my life. "Drink the pain and responsibilities away; you know how to do that well."

The reasonable side of my brain—my realistic self-talk—said, "But you could end up just like him."

My alcohol-saturated brain replied, "I don't care. Have another drink."

That battle, the one that started right there in the bar, ultimately lasted two more years—two more arduous years of letting myself down. After that, I finally mustered the courage to confront the consequences of my actions and visited the doctor to assess the damage I had caused myself. The prospect of what they might find was terrifying. I anticipated that the blood tests would reveal elevated levels of liver enzymes, indicative of abnormal liver function, which was just one of the many horrifying outcomes I was expecting. And indeed, the tests indicated exactly what I feared. It was a stark wake-up call, signaling that it was well beyond time to take decisive action. I created a new affirmation and mantra: "I am stronger than this, and my future is worth it."

I *never* thought that I would be where I am today, and I want to share the miracle roadmap that got me here with others who know the same struggles I do. This book, *Free Yourself from the Grip of Alcohol Addiction*, was born from that pivotal moment in my life and the ensuing journey I started as a result. This guide isn't just a set of instructions for breaking free from the clutches of alcohol; it's a testament to my personal fight against the bindings of alcohol addiction, shared with you. It puts me in a very vulnerable place to share this with you, to share these intimate details of my life, but I'm doing so because within these pages lies a promise—a promise of renewal and strength, a promise that sobriety isn't just a dream but a reachable, maintainable reality.

My path was rickety and not-so-clear, which isn't the journey that I want you to have. For that reason, I've structured this guide into 10 clear, actionable steps, each enlightened by the personal experiences that shaped my path to sobriety. Inside, you'll find those personal experiences intertwined with scientific, psychological research to help you discover your own personal path to healing. It's designed to resonate with anyone—no matter your background or how heavy your struggles with alcohol may feel. I know as well as you do that alcoholism isn't just about putting down the bottle; it's about understanding why we hold it so tightly in the first place and how we can let go, rebuild, and flourish. I've poured every lesson learned, every setback, and every victory into these pages to create a guide and companion for your journey to sobriety.

As you turn these pages, remember that if I was able to make it to sobriety, you can, too. Please take this as an opportunity to do more than read—to reflect, write, and apply these steps in your life with the knowledge that you, too, are worth it. The best way to approach this guide is with an open heart and a resolve to change. No journey to sobriety is free of struggles, but with every step forward, you're moving closer to a life that's full of health, wellness, and fulfillment. It's a life you *deserve,* not just some fairytale.

Start this journey not just with the hope of quitting alcohol but to transform your entire life. Along the way, you will enhance your mental and physical well-being, forge stronger relationships, and rebuild your self-confidence; it all starts now.

So, here we are at the beginning of something profound. This book is your first step in reaching sobriety and changing your life. With each chapter and story shared, know that a fulfilling, sober life isn't just possible—it's within your reach right here and now. Let's step forward together with hope, courage, and the strong belief that we can overcome more than we ever thought possible.

STEP #1

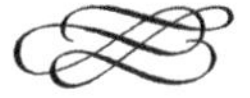

THE REALITY OF ALCOHOL ADDICTION

More times than I would like to admit, I've found myself sitting alone, peering into the empty bottom of a glass and wondering how every single moment of my life led to that occasion. If you've ever experienced this, you're far from alone. Alcohol addiction is more common than people think, with more than 15 million people in the United States alone suffering from it (*Alcoholism Statistics You Need to Know*, 2018). Fighting something like this starts with understanding, and understanding alcohol addiction is more than just knowing that you should probably drink less. In order to manage alcohol addiction, you also have to understand the science of how alcohol addiction impacts your brain and reels you in, as well as how it affects your life more broadly. So, let's start by exploring some brainy stuff that can help you understand why quitting feels so hard but is entirely achievable nonetheless.

THE SCIENCE OF ADDICTION: HOW ALCOHOL REWIRES YOUR BRAIN

Addiction happens because of the ability of a substance—in our case, alcohol—to rewire your brain. You know that warm, fuzzy feeling you get after you take the first sip of your favorite drink? That's your brain's reward system kicking into high gear. Alcohol floods your brain with dopamine, the "feel-good" neurotransmitter, creating a shortcut to pleasure with a single sip. In this way, alcohol takes advantage of something called neurological pathways in the brain, which operate kind of like roads, allowing alcohol to drive its way into your brain directly. Over time, your brain starts relying on alcohol-induced dopamine spikes to feel happy, making it a challenge to find enjoyment in less stimulating, everyday activities such as your hobbies or relaxation. This means that alcohol can go beyond just a craving for a drink and into the territory of a *need,* at least where your neurology is concerned.

Beyond dopamine, alcohol throws a wrench into the works of other neurotransmitters—chemicals that help regulate everything from your mood to how well you sleep (Cleveland Clinic, 2022a). Regular drinking can decrease the levels of serotonin that your brain produces. Because serotonin helps regulate your mood, the disruption of serotonin transmitters because of alcohol addiction can lead to anxiety and depression. Alcohol addiction can also mess with GABA, a neurotransmitter that helps control impulsiveness, in turn making you more likely to make poor decisions after a few drinks (Cleveland Clinic, 2022b). This chemical chaos means that you may struggle with regulating emotions, mood, motivation, and more, which also worsens your dependency on alcohol as your brain attempts to manage this chaos.

Additionally, alcohol addiction can result in cognitive decline. For example, have you ever had trouble remembering what you did the morning after a few drinks? That's because alcohol can impair your hippocampus, the part of your brain responsible for making memories (Wendt, 2022). Regularly drinking in large quantities can lead to more permanent slips in memory and even affect your ability to make sound decisions. Just like driving through fog, where everything is slower and it's hard to see where you're going, the cognitive impairment of alcohol addiction can make life a bit foggy. This cognitive fog makes it even harder to make the positive changes needed to overcome addiction.

Despite all of this, there is some good news: Your brain is somewhat of a superhero in that it can heal and rewire itself, a phenomenon known as neuroplasticity. This means that, despite the damage from alcohol, your brain can start to repair itself with sustained sobriety. Over time, the fog of alcohol addiction lifts, memories sharpen, and the balance in neurotransmitter levels can be restored. Recovery gives your brain a chance to return to a healthier, happier state.

THE EFFECTS OF ALCOHOL ADDICTION: HEALTH, RELATIONSHIPS, AND MORE

At first, it's easy to think that alcoholism only impacts you and that those impacts aren't that severe. Beyond impacting the brain's basic functions, addiction can affect physical health, mental health, and even the relationships you have with others in severe ways. Understanding these impacts is helpful in recovery, allowing you to correct the harm caused to others and to yourself through addiction.

Physical Health and Alcohol: A Tale of Harm and Recovery

Let's be real about our insides for a moment—specifically, how alcohol has been throwing a not-so-silent party in there, and trust me; it's not the fun kind. Drinking alcohol, especially in excess, is like sending an unruly party guest through your body, and this guest isn't respectful of your space. It barges through vital organs like the liver, heart, and pancreas, often leaving a trail of damage behind. The liver, bless its hard-working soul, gets the brunt of it. It's your body's detoxifier, constantly filtering out the bad stuff. But alcohol? That's a whole different level of evil, and over time, the liver gets overwhelmed—it starts to scar, resulting in something called cirrhosis, and the liver's ability to fight off toxins diminishes (*Alcoholic Liver Disease Information,* n.d.). This doesn't even take into account the heart, which has to pump harder as alcohol messes with your blood pressure, leading to potential long-term heart diseases. There's also the pancreas, often forgotten, which gets inflamed, leading to pancreatitis—which is as painful as it sounds.

Now, if that internal house party sounds chaotic, just wait until you hear about your immune system—or what's left of it after regular drinking. Alcohol tricks your body, making it feel invincible when it comes to stress. But when the body faces a stressor like an infection, the promises of alcohol are nowhere to be found. Alcohol leaves your immune system weak and thus leaves you more susceptible to illness (Sarkar, Jung, & Wang, 2015). From a common cold to an infection, you are vulnerable, all because your immune system's guards are down thanks to alcohol consumption.

Alcohol's Shadow on Mental Health: Anxiety, Depression, and Beyond

Alcohol is tricky in that it wriggles into your life, promising to be the life of the party, the comforter, the stress-buster, yet it only offers these things for a short amount of time. Shortly after you invite alcohol into your life, it makes a mess of things—stressing you out *more,* causing more pain, and creating more trouble than it's worth. The dangerous, backstabbing effects of alcohol are the reason that there is such a significant link between alcohol addiction and mental health disorders, often referred to as dual diagnosis (Alcohol and Drug Foundation, 2021). This effect goes beyond a rough day and needing a drink to relax, creating ongoing battles with disorders like anxiety or depression in addition to addiction.

Managing alcohol addiction along with the resultant mental health concerns that follow is a self-fulfilling prophecy, where one issue feeds into and exacerbates the other. Alcohol is often used at first to self-medicate mental anguish, but it eventually intensifies the symptoms it was meant to alleviate. This creates a vicious cycle that's tough to break. Then, just when you think you've experienced the worst of it, anxiety brings along its friend depression and takes things to a new level of terrible. This cycle can feel like being stuck on a merry-go-round you can't jump off, spinning out of control.

Getting out of this cycle is no easy pursuit. It requires a holistic approach where your mental health receives as much attention as your sobriety. Recovery is more robust when the roots of mental distress are addressed, especially considering that emotional distress can be a major trigger for cravings and relapse. If you're only fixing the leaks in your roof but ignoring your house's crumbling foundation, you'll be under a collapse. Sobriety might patch the leaks, but understanding and treating your mental health shores up the foundation.

The Ripple Effect: How Your Drinking Affects Loved Ones

When you throw a rock into a river, the ripples span the entire surface of the water, not just the space around the rock. Alcohol addiction is like that. It doesn't just affect you; your family, friends, and colleagues are all involved, too, feeling the ripples from your actions. It's tough to admit, but our battles with alcohol don't just affect us—they splash onto everyone around us, often more dramatically than we might realize while we're in the thick of it.

The strain that alcohol addiction places on your relationships is no joke. Friends and family members often feel constantly let down by those with an addiction, as the addiction often leads to choosing alcohol over your friends and family over and over. One drink turns into five, and suddenly, you can't go out to that birthday dinner or help your friend move like you promised. Over time, these broken plans and unmet expectations start to erode trust. Family dinners, essential conversations with your partner, work commitments—these can all start to feel the strain of unpredictability and disappointment from alcoholism. Every drink adds weight to a scale, and eventually, something's got to give.

The emotional toll that your addiction has on loved ones is massive. Your loved ones are likely to experience a roller-coaster of hope and despair—up when you're doing well, down when you're not. They worry, get angry and sad, and often feel helpless because they feel like they can't help pull you back from the edge of addiction. The stress of watching someone suffer and being unable to help can lead to anxiety and depression in your loved ones. They may even feel anger over the fact that you are unable to recognize the effects of your addiction on your life and theirs.

Alcohol addiction can also be worsened through social relationships because of something called enabling. Enabling is where a loved one might try to help you cope or heal, but it actually makes your addiction worse by allowing you to continue to drink without consequences (Cohen, 2022). For example, your spouse calling in sick because you're hungover means that you can continue to rely on this "support," when in reality, they are just smoothing things over. It's done with the best intentions, and you usually aren't responsible for someone deciding to enable you, but enabling reinforces the behavior it tries to mitigate. This can be tiring for both you and your loved ones, causing further tension.

At one point, the guilt of how my addiction affected my loved ones overwhelmed me. I felt like the worst person on Earth, and the shame consumed me. However, during my recovery, I realized something. When it comes to healing the broken or damaged social bonds of addiction, you have to be mindful that guilt and shame might set in, but those emotions shouldn't take hold. Feeling guilty won't change the past; only your dedication can. Rather than ruminating, it's important to find a way forward that balances taking responsibility alongside working to heal those bonds as you recover.

Healing these rifts and rebuilding healthier dynamics doesn't happen overnight and certainly doesn't happen in a vacuum. It involves open, honest conversations where you listen to how your behavior has impacted those around you. This also means acknowledging the feelings of your loved ones without immediately jumping to your defense. It is always tempting to do that—to try and defend oneself in the face of perceived judgment—but talking about your own feelings should never be a rebuttal to someone else's.

Beyond that, this process includes setting boundaries together, where you and your loved ones understand what behaviors are no longer acceptable and the consequences if those boundaries are crossed. Cooperation and support have to flow in both directions—them supporting your journey to sobriety and you respecting the emotional boundaries they need to maintain their mental health—for these bonds to be repaired.

In this rebuilding phase, transparency is your most valuable tool. You have to be upfront with your struggles, successes, and setbacks as you recover. You can achieve this by allowing your loved ones to celebrate with you when you hit a milestone and letting them in when you find things challenging. This shared journey can bring you closer and create a new level of trust and understanding. It transforms the dynamic from one of dependency and frustration to one of mutual support and respect.

ACTIVITIES FOR FORWARD MOTION

Now that you have a bit of understanding regarding alcohol addiction and how it impacts you, let's take a look at two activities that can help you get started on your journey.

Reflecting on Your Brain Health

If a friend were to borrow your car and then return it with dents and engine problems, you'd be pretty quick to fix it, right? You wouldn't wait to act until it was convenient because your car is important—it's a symbol and a daily need alike. Now, think of your brain like that car. Alcohol has been rough on it, sure, but it's not beyond repair. Considering your recovery like this can sometimes make all the difference in motivating you to stick to your sobriety goals. So many people think that all hope is lost, but that is far from the case. It just takes some care, consideration, and mindful repairs to return your mind to a state of health.

With this in mind, achieving your goals can be easier if you have a strong idea of what it is you hope to achieve through recovery. Jot down how you feel mentally right now and what changes you would like to see during the process of recovery. As you write about your current state and your goals moving forward, keep in mind that sobriety is not just about becoming alcohol-free (AF)—it's about striving for a healthier, clearer-minded version of yourself.

Creating a Personal Mantra

A personal mantra is a statement or question that you can use to remind yourself of your goals and aspirations. My mantra guided me through my darkest times: "Was that drink and fake feeling of that drink worth risking your life?" Each and every time I repeated this question to myself, my answer was a resounding, "No way!" This becomes clearer every day of my journey, and it will be for you as well.

For this activity, take a pause to create your empowering mantras for self-encouragement. Ponder on affirmations that strike a chord within you and commit them to paper, ideally in a journal or another place where you can reference them often. Some mantras that you can use for yourself or adapt to your needs include:

- I deserve to feel happy and healthy and to be addiction-free.
- Addiction is not stronger than I am. I can beat this.
- I am worth the dedication and effort of sobriety.

The powerful mantras you create will become your best friends during the recovery process, steering you toward a state of clarity and abstinence. As you progress toward recovery, remember that it's okay to revise your mantras. What works for you now might not work a year into your recovery, and it's absolutely okay to modify your mantras as needed.

The reality of alcohol addiction is severe, and understanding that is step one in the process of freeing yourself from the grips of alcohol addiction. Alcohol addiction can creep into every area of your life, and healing from that requires a multipronged approach where you balance repairing relationships with others alongside what you need to heal, inside and out. As we close off this chapter, remember that alcohol addiction isn't some massive cement wall that you're unable to bust through; it's a gate, and finding the key to unlock the path to sobriety relies on your conscious effort. One way to get closer to finding that key is by dismantling myths behind alcoholism.

STEP #2

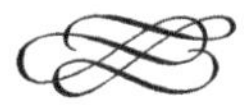

UNDERSTANDING ALCOHOLISM THROUGH MYTHS VS. FACTS

Part of recovery involves understanding alcohol addiction, and digging deeper to improve that understanding is our second step. Alcohol consumption is surrounded by dozens of misconceptions—myths that drive people to keep drinking because they provide excuses or pose barriers to recovery. For example, have you ever heard someone brag about being a "functional alcoholic" like it's a badge of honor? It's almost as if they're saying, "Look at me; I can drink like a fish and still hold down a job and my life!" This is just one of the many myths that surrounds alcohol addiction and makes it harder to truly recover. As the second step toward your healing, let's unpack some of the myths that contribute to alcohol addiction and discover the true facts behind these myths.

MYTH #1: THE "FUNCTIONAL ALCOHOLIC"

So, you think you're a functional alcoholic because you've never been fired or because your family hasn't disowned you? I get it. I've been there, using my responsibilities as an excuse against the truth of my addiction. I felt like if I was working and balancing things well, then it didn't matter how much I drank. However, there is a critical distinction to make here—functioning does not equate to flourishing.

Many believe that as long as they're handling their responsibilities, their drinking isn't a problem. Sure, I wasn't being fired, and my family hadn't caught on yet, but calling myself a functional alcoholic overlooked the silent battles I was experiencing: The morning headaches, the guilt, and the mental gymnastics to justify the last drink and the next. You might feel like you're doing just fine, but there's a difference between appearing fine to others and functioning. If you're battling yourself just like I was or trying to justify drinking or its effects, then you're *not* functional at all; you just wear a good mask.

Then Long-Term Consequences of Feigning "Functional"

While that mask might feel like your saving grace, it's not without consequences. Maintaining a façade of functionality can work for a while, but it's a bit like duct-taping a leaky pipe. The tape holds for now, but that pressure is building up, and eventually, it will burst. The long-term consequences of trying to front as a functional alcoholic sneak up on you. We're talking about health issues that range from liver disease to heart problems, anxiety, and depression. Relationships can also suffer—what seems manageable now can gradually erode your closest connections, just like we talked about earlier. Career impacts might not be immediate, but the cumulative effects of too many late starts, missed deadlines, or lackluster performances start to add up as well. Worst of all, you might *think* that you're doing fine, but when it comes to alcoholism, everyone *around* you can tell that something is up. By the time you realize how deep you are, you're not functioning; you're floundering.

The Danger of Denial

Denial is the bedrock of the functional alcoholic myth. It whispers, "You're doing just fine," while you ignore the warning signs. This denial is dangerous because it delays the help and intervention needed to recover, often until things spiral beyond control. The longer you ignore the problem, the harder it becomes to address it. Denial isn't just a river in Egypt; it keeps you wading deeper into troubled waters.

Path to Recovery

Admitting you have a problem doesn't make you weak; it makes you honest. Starting on the path to recovery begins with dropping the façade of functionality and facing the facts. This involves recognizing that you don't have to wait for your life to fall apart before putting it back together. Recovery is not for the faint-hearted. It's tough, messy, and probably one of the bravest things you'll ever do. But it starts with acknowledging that just because you're managing doesn't mean you're thriving. From there, you can begin taking steps toward a life where you survive and live in your newly created, exciting world.

Reflect and Write: Are You Really "Just Fine?"

If you're ready to examine your drinking habits seriously, grab a notebook and write down your answers to these questions. You can use the same notebook for all the exercises in this book, creating a recovery journal. As you answer these questions, be brutally honest with yourself—doing so is the first step toward genuine change.

1. What responsibilities do you use to convince yourself that drinking isn't a problem?
2. List some subtle ways your life has been impacted by alcohol that you might be overlooking.
3. What lies or half-truths are you telling yourself about your drinking habits or their consequences?

You don't have to judge yourself here. The point of journaling about these things is to have a conversation with yourself that will lead to a healthier, happier you.

MYTH #2: DRINKING IN MODERATION (IT RARELY WORKS FOR ADDICTS)

Moderation is a sticky trap that many addicts get caught in. It starts like this: You've decided to cut down on your drinking—just a couple of drinks a night, nothing major. Sounds reasonable, right? You're still in control and have everything handled, so there's no reason to worry. But then, a stressful day at work, a fight with your partner, or even a celebration comes up, and suddenly, those two drinks turn into three, four, or more. Before you know it, moderation seems like a joke your brain played on you. If this feels familiar to you, it's because addiction isn't something you can manage in moderation. Someone who is addicted to something can't enjoy it just a little bit because the brain is hardwired to go into overdrive at the smallest amount of the substance. One drink behind the guise of moderation is often a slippery slope into spiraling, as it makes the brain crave more and more.

The crux of the problem for many people with an addiction lies in the fundamental misunderstanding of addiction versus control. Addiction is not a failure of will or a lapse in moral judgment—it has nothing to do with how well you can engage moderately. Rather, addiction is a deep-seated disorder that alters how your brain processes pleasure, pain, reward, and risk. When you tell yourself you'll only drink in moderation, you're essentially trying to negotiate with a brain that's been rewired for compulsion. Your brain might concede to just a drink or two now, but soon, it will be begging for more, and in an attempt to quell its tantrums for more, you will give in. This is why moderation has no place in recovery.

When you try to facilitate a relationship with a substance that hinges on moderation, you also open the door to cravings—an insatiable thirst, no pun intended, to turn to the bottle over and over. Cravings don't care about your plans for moderation. They are born from a physiological need—your brain's demand for dopamine or an evening free from the day-to-day stress that is becoming too much to bear. These cravings can make the idea of just one drink laughable because they're not playing by the logical rules of moderation. Instead, they're playing by the no-holds-barred rules of addiction. Each time you give in to these cravings, it reinforces the cycle, making the next craving even more intense. This, in turn, creates a feedback loop that's as exhausting as it is destructive. During the height of my addiction, I often found myself trapped in a relentless downward spiral that was enforced by trying to seek moderation when what I really needed was abstinence. The question, "Why can't I achieve that moderation?" lingered.

These reasons are why, for many people struggling with alcohol dependency, abstinence—not moderation—tends to be the most effective approach. If touching a hot stove burns your hand, you don't keep touching it with fewer fingers, hoping it'll hurt less—you stop touching it altogether. Recovering from addiction is just like that. While harm reduction can control some of the damage, you're still being burned regardless. Moreover, numerous studies and countless personal stories back the idea of abstinence up, showing that removing alcohol entirely cuts off the feedback loop of craving and indulgence, giving your brain a chance to heal and build new, healthier pathways (Eddie et al., 2022).

Planning for Wellness: Setting Small Goals

It can be hard to wake up one day and decide to go cold turkey, especially if you're physically dependent on alcohol. Taking it one small step at a time with the ultimate end goal of abstinence can help you fight the monster that is addiction. Doing so requires you to set and stick to realistic goals. Aiming for sobriety means recognizing that moderation is a temporary stepping stone, not a final destination.

To set small and realistic goals that help you begin the process, start with manageable, measurable objectives—such as joining a support group and talking to a counselor and doctor. When I started the process, I used moderation as a first step to ultimate abstinence by challenging myself to spend a single weekend sober. It didn't seem like a lot to those around me, but for me, that was a huge victory. One weekend turned into several weeks in a row, which ultimately led me to where I am today.

Use these victories—big or small—as a foundation to set more ambitious goals, like exploring new interests that aren't linked to drinking, mending relationships affected by alcohol, and pursuing both personal and professional achievements that were previously obstructed by drinking. This approach doesn't mean that you are preparing for failure, but rather that you're being aware of potential setbacks and giving yourself the best opportunity to avoid them.

MYTH #3: ALCOHOLICS SIMPLY DON'T WANT TO QUIT

There's this prevailing belief that alcoholics are addicted simply because they don't want to quit. People wrongly believe that it's related to being lazy or a failure when the reality is that alcoholism is a *disease.* Alcoholism isn't a badge of failure or a sign that someone simply doesn't want to give up on drinking. It's a medical condition, a mental illness, and a disease that has nothing to do with "not wanting" to heal. In fact, many alcoholics desire nothing more than to heal. And besides, any disease requires careful treatment and isn't something that can be "fixed" overnight. No one tells a person with diabetes to "get over" their need for insulin, a life-saving medical intervention, so why do people expect someone with alcoholism to quit drinking magically through sheer willpower alone?

The medical perspective surrounding alcohol addiction—which includes understanding the physiological nature of addiction—is crucial not just for those struggling with the addiction but also for everyone around them. When you start understanding alcoholism as a disease, it shifts how you approach everything, from treatment to day-to-day interactions. It means getting the right kind of help—medical interventions, therapy, support groups—without the added burden of guilt or blame. It also shifts the mindset surrounding alcohol addiction to managing a condition, not condemning a character. When we emphasize that alcoholism is a disease, we no longer see ourselves as failures but as people who are dealing with a health issue that needs attention and care.

Shifting mindsets surrounding addiction can be life-changing as well because it removes the stigma that makes it hard for many to seek help—something that played a huge role in why I didn't seek help sooner. Stigma is the prevailing attitude about something, usually stemming from a place of judgment. The stigma surrounding addiction creates fear in addicts, and the fear of being judged or labeled as an addict can keep you from feeling safe reaching out, locking you in a cycle of silence and drinking. It's heartbreaking. It can also compel you to hide your struggle, dodge treatment, or worse, lose hope. Changing the narrative around alcoholism is how we can begin to dismantle the stigma, and it starts with conversations like this one. We have to talk openly and honestly about alcoholism for what it is: a complex health issue.

Battling stigma and the myth that alcoholics are failures or lazy isn't easy, but sharing your story and advocating for the education of others can be a lot of help. People understand things more readily through a first-hand perspective; it's why I'm sharing my story with you. When someone understands alcoholism and addiction more clearly, instead of just leafing through scientific literature about it, they can connect to the story and the person behind it with greater empathy. Sharing your story is a big step toward dismantling the hush-hush attitude people have about addiction. Likewise, it's so important to encourage people to become educated about the nature of addiction. No one *wants* to be addicted; they want to be pain-free, and helping others understand that fights off this myth once and for all.

MYTH #4: ALCOHOL WITHDRAWAL ISN'T *THAT* BAD!

A lot of people are afraid of going sober because they don't want to deal with withdrawals, and people who don't know what it's like will say things like, "It can't be *that* bad," in response. Withdrawal is more than just the world's worst hangover. When you decide to break up with alcohol, especially if it's been a long-term, heavy relationship, your body can throw a bit of a fit. Withdrawal isn't just painful—it can also be dangerous if not handled tactfully. Like any breakup, it will hurt before it gets better, but understanding what you're up against can make the process less daunting, and it starts with overcoming this fourth myth about alcohol addiction.

The Reality of Withdrawal

Let's start with the symptoms of alcohol withdrawal. Physically, you might feel like you've been hit by a truck—headaches, nausea, shaking, sweating, and even fever are common (Mary Jo DiLonardo, 2010). These sensations are your body's way of adjusting to the absence of its usual chemical chaos. Psychologically, it can be just as challenging, if not tougher. You might experience anxiety, irritability, or mood swings. Sleep might elude you, and, in more severe cases, there can be hallucinations or seizures. It's not pretty, but it's important to remember that these symptoms are a sign of your body regaining its equilibrium. It might be scary to even hear about this, but you have to remember that not only is it different for each person, but the withdrawal symptoms are well worth it for the reward of regaining your health.

The timeline of the symptoms of withdrawal can vary widely from person to person. The acute withdrawal phase can typically last anywhere from a few days to around two weeks, starting from the time you stop drinking (Casali, 2021). The first 48 hours are usually the toughest. This is when you're more likely to experience the most intense physical symptoms, as your body is taking the biggest hits from the changes sparked by putting down the bottle. After that, you might start feeling physically better, but the psychological grip can linger. This is what's often referred to as PAWS, or post-acute withdrawal syndrome, where symptoms like anxiety, low mood, and sleep disturbances can continue for months (*Post-Acute-Withdrawal Syndrome (PAWS): An In-Depth Guide*, 2018). It's a marathon, not a sprint, and preparing yourself for this can help you manage expectations and stay committed to your sobriety path.

In some cases, attaining sobriety might require something called medical detoxification. The fact that medical detox enters the equation only solidifies how serious withdrawal can be; it's no laughing matter. Going cold turkey can be dangerous without proper medical supervision, especially if you've been a heavy drinker. Medical detox is often thought to be something people do solely for comfort during the withdrawal process, but it's not just a comfort thing; it's a matter of safety. In a detox facility, medical professionals can monitor your symptoms and administer medications to help ease the process and reduce the risk of severe complications like seizures, which is why you should never feel ashamed to consider a medical detox if you need or want it.

As we wrap up this chapter, remember that understanding the process of overcoming alcohol addiction is multifaceted. It involves understanding the reality behind some of the biggest myths people believe, as well as the fact that stigma shouldn't be a barrier to your healing, no matter what others think of you or your process. Beyond that, knowing what symptoms to expect, how long they might last, and the importance of medical supervision means that you're better equipped to handle this challenging phase.

Now, it's time to build on this foundational knowledge, exploring strategies for long-term sobriety and how to integrate new, healthier habits into your life. The road to recovery is not just about removing alcohol from your life; it starts with motivation.

STEP #3

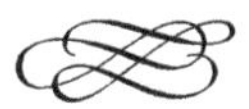

BUILDING YOUR MOTIVATION

Have you ever daydreamed about a life where your first thought isn't about whether it's too early for a drink? Or perhaps you've envisioned a morning where you wake up energized, your head clear, and your day is not planned around your next drink? I sure have. It's these flickers of a life not dictated by alcohol that start to sow the seeds of motivation. But let's take that further—transform those flickers into a blazing trail of change. This chapter—step three of your journey—is about stoking that fire of motivation, taking your vision of sobriety beyond dreams and into reality.

VISUALIZING YOUR LIFE WITHOUT ALCOHOL: A JOURNEY OF REDISCOVERY

Sometimes, the very inspiration for making a massive change can be found within your own mind. Imagining a sober future is the start of the process, where your aspirations and "one day" thoughts become the path to day one of sobriety. This involves visualizing, setting visual-based goals, and even allowing the success stories of others to inspire you.

The Power of Visualization

Picture this: It's six months from now, and you've been sober the entire time. You wake up in the morning feeling refreshed, not wrecked. Your day is a new beginning, where you don't have to plan out each movement. Instead, you can enjoy the hard work you've put in and spend time doing what you love. You feel at peace. This isn't a pipe dream; it's a genuine possibility that you can create for yourself as you move toward a sober life.

If you didn't actually "picture" the above, I would like you to take a moment to do so. Truly visualize what your life might look like six months from now if you start this journey today. I bet it feels exciting, and maybe even scary (in a good way), to be able to live alcohol-free. The reason that I wanted you to really "see" that life is because of the power of visualization in striking motivation.

Visualizing your life without alcohol isn't like waving a magic wand and pretending everything is perfect. Instead, visualization allows you to see all the potential joys and achievements that lie hidden under the fog of alcohol. Through visualization, your mind can paint a picture so compelling that you're magnetically drawn to it, motivated by the real benefits of sobriety. Whether reconnecting with old hobbies, discovering new passions, or simply enjoying the clarity of waking up without a hangover, each image you create is a step toward making those visualizations a reality.

Visualizing the future you want to have is an incredible first step in gaining motivation.

Benefits Beyond Health

While the health benefits of quitting alcohol are vast and vital, the perks of sobriety spill over into every corner of your life. Being aware of the benefits beyond health can serve as further inspiration for your recovery. For example, sobriety can allow relationships to transform and deepen when they no longer operate based on your drinking habits. Your career and personal projects can flourish when they get the full force of your attention and creativity. Think about it —every ounce of energy and time you spend thinking about, acquiring, and consuming alcohol is now yours to redirect. Where could that energy take you? Perhaps it's advancing your career, picking up an old college hobby, or even starting a new relationship based on honesty and presence. Sobriety is the key to adding layers of richness to your life that were previously drowned out. It's important to keep this in mind as a part of your journey.

Setting Vision-Based Goals

It's not enough, however, to just visualize. These visions must be turned into real, actionable goals to make them stick. Vague resolutions like "drink less" or "be healthier" don't count either; you have to make specific, vision-based goals directly tied to the sober life you're imagining. Want to wake up feeling refreshed? Set a goal to establish a calming nighttime routine. Are you dreaming of picking up your guitar again? Set a goal to play a little daily, or maybe take lessons. These goals should be clear and linked directly to your sobriety's benefits, making them desirable and achievable. They're the signposts on your road to recovery, guiding you, step-by-step, to the life you've envisioned.

Success Stories as Inspiration

Sometimes, seeing is believing. Hearing from those who've traveled this road before can be incredibly inspiring. For example, when I was starting my journey to sobriety, I always looked up to my friend John. John found that after six months of sobriety, he could start a small business—something he'd always dreamed of but never had the clarity or energy to pursue while drinking. Someone else who I looked up to was my co-worker's wife, Tammy, who rekindled her love for painting and held her first gallery showing a year into her sobriety. And most significantly, there's me, who aspired to guide others toward the illuminating path of sobriety, showing how it can transform your world. Had I ever envisioned myself as the author of a book? No! But now, that vision has become a reality for me. It was not easy or inexpensive, but if I can help even just one person, my goal is accomplished and my heart is brighter.

Looking up to others as a part of your journey can help prove to yourself that your path leads to places you may have thought were mapped only in dreams. Right now, take out your notebook or journal you were working with earlier. Write down three to five people who you can look up to for inspiration on your journey. You can include:

- People you know personally, like friends and family
- People you've read about or seen on TV, either real people or characters
- Celebrities who have become sober
- Anyone else whose path resembles or inspires your own in some way

In moments of challenge, when it seems like the path is too hard to bear, you can think of these inspirational people and visualize your success from the basis of theirs.

Reflect on Your Potential

Finally, it's time to reflect on your potential when it comes to recovery. You can grab your journal or just a scrap of paper and jot down some answers:

- What would you do if alcohol no longer controlled your day?
- What passions would you explore?
- Who might you reconnect with?

Write it down, make it feel tangible, and then step back and look at all you could gain. The possibilities for your life are boundless when recovery is involved.

SETTING INTENTIONS: THE ROLE OF PERSONAL GOALS IN SOBRIETY

Building your motivation for recovery also relies on setting intentions for your journey in the form of personal goals. Let's dive into the heart of setting intentions because, honestly, even the best explorers can get lost without a map. Setting clear, specific, and measurable goals doesn't just involve ticking boxes or making nice lists—it's a method that involves giving your sobriety journey direction and purpose. Think of it this way: If sobriety is your destination, your goals are the milestones along the way. They keep you on track, motivated, and clear about where you're headed and why it's worth the trip.

The thing about goals is that they need to be as transparent as the sky on a sunny day. Vague goals are like fog; they obscure the path and make it easy to wander off course. So, if you want to "drink less," how do you know when you've achieved that? Instead, a goal like "attend three support meetings per week" or "spend two nights a week at a hobby class instead of at the bar" gives you a clear target. It's tangible, measurable, and, most importantly, actionable. Each checkmark on that list is a step forward, a tangible sign of your progress that motivates you and gives you something to look back on and say, "I did that," when the going gets tough.

My Journey With Sobriety Goals

To illustrate the power of setting tangible goals for myself, I crafted a personal list for the upcoming year designed to enrich my life beyond sobriety. This list included embarking on a cruise, trekking to Hanging Lake in Glenwood Springs, experiencing the thrill of skydiving, attending three outdoor concerts, decluttering my space, mastering the art of healthy cooking—a passion of mine that made this goal more enjoyable—participating in a company golf tournament, and achieving a healthier weight by addressing the pounds accumulated from drinking. This last goal was more attainable than anticipated; cutting out alcohol paved the way for a natural progression toward a healthier weight. The result was a significant loss of 40 pounds. Setting goals that align with what you visualized earlier—goals that are tangible and actionable—is an amazing way to build motivation and catapult yourself forward in your journey.

Short-Term Goals Matter

For a lot of people, it's tempting to jump right in with big goals for sobriety and improving life; for others, this can be daunting. The good news is that instead of picking one of the other, you can—and should—find a combination of both long- and short-term goals that work for you. Short-term goals are your immediate focus, crafting momentum through daily or weekly achievements that offer quick wins and continuous motivation. In contrast, long-term goals represent the distant horizon—constantly visible yet far-reaching. These are your overarching aspirations, the significant life alterations you aim to realize through sobriety, whether mending a crucial relationship or reaching a professional landmark.

Both goal types are interconnected; the victories of short-term goals fuel your daily motivation, whereas long-term goals provide a clear direction and significant objectives to pursue. I recommend setting three long-term and three short-term goals to get yourself started out on a foot of motivation. Why wait? Jot down some goals for yourself now —or after you finish this chapter so that you don't miss out on helpful tips.

Aligning Your Goals With Values

Aligning your goals with your values is where the magic happens when it comes to goals. This alignment turns goals from a "must do" into a "want to do." I mean, think about it. How many times have you set a goal and, because it felt like a chore, forgot all about it? Aligning your goals with your values prevents this from happening. When you align your goals with your values, it helps connect your objectives to what truly matters to you. For example, if family is a core value to you, try to set goals that enhance your relationships and family time. Passionate about creativity? Aim to start a project or revisit an old hobby that alcohol has pushed aside. This connection energizes you and embeds your goals deeply into your path, making them part of your identity and dreams rather than just tasks on a list.

Celebrate Success, Big or Small

Acknowledging and celebrating each step of your journey is crucial to maintaining motivation. Small goals might not seem like much, but rewarding and treating yourself for each small victory can be helpful in maintaining much-needed motivation. You might celebrate a week sober with a movie night or a month sober by buying yourself a new outfit.

My path to sobriety began with a simple act: Encircling the number 1 on a calendar to represent my first day without alcohol. This act became a ritual, with each subsequent day gaining its own circle, creating a chain of consecutive victories. It's easy to forget how far you've come, especially on the days that most test your resolve. Keeping a progress journal or using a visual tool, like marking off each sober day on a calendar like I did, can reinforce your commitment.

In setting these goals, remember that the path of sobriety is uniquely yours. Your goals should reflect your journey by being tailored to your needs, challenges, and dreams. So, set them with intention, pursue them with passion, and let them lead you to the life you've envisioned—one sober day at a time.

THE POWER OF WHY: IDENTIFYING YOUR REASONS FOR QUITTING DRINKING

When it comes to keeping yourself motivated, understanding why you want to quit drinking in the first place can be a big help. I mean, have you ever caught yourself in the middle of a task, sweating and hustling, and suddenly paused to ask yourself, "Wait, why am I even doing this?" It's quite the stopper. Well, wrestling the beast that is alcohol addiction isn't much different. Understanding your deep-seated reasons for wanting to quit can be your anchor, even when relapse calls your name.

That said, let's dig into the "why" of your sobriety. Grab your journal and find a quiet corner because it's time to have a heart-to-heart with yourself. Start by writing down all the reasons you can think of for why you want to stop drinking, even if you repeat the reasons from earlier prompts I've provided. Don't overthink it; just let the reasons flow. Done? Great. Now go through that list and ask yourself, "Is this my voice or someone else's? Is this a deep-rooted personal desire or something I feel pressured into?" Part of this exercise is about distinguishing reasons that truly belong to you from the pressures of external expectations, which can be demotivating. This will aid in helping you find your own authentic why.

The brilliance of having a strong, personal why is its power to guide you through the stormiest parts of your sobriety. When a craving hits or a setback blindsides you, what will make you dig your heels in and say, "No, I'm sticking with my choice?" A nebulous, external reason like "because I'm supposed to" will not cut it. But is there a reason that has to do with what *you* want for yourself? That's a banner you can rally behind. It becomes your mantra—your battle cry in the face of challenges—and you should let those powerful internal reasons be your reason for sobriety.

With your goals in mind, it can still be easy for self-doubt to creep in and make you feel uncertain. That's precisely why revisiting and reinforcing your thinking regularly is critical. For this, I recommend making it a habit—weekly or monthly, depending on your preferences—to reflect on your motivations with each new sobriety milestone and goal you set. For example, you can ask yourself if your goals have changed in any way or if your values have strengthened. Knowing where your why begins and ends will keep you motivated beyond just today.

FROM FEAR TO COURAGE: OVERCOMING THE ANXIETY OF CHANGE

The thought of life without alcohol can be terrifying, especially if alcohol has been your best friend for the longest time. That fear you're feeling about giving it up? It's normal. It's your brain's way of protecting you from the unknown, waving red flags and screaming, "Hey, are you sure about this?" Everyone experiences this anxiety when confronted with a pretty major lifestyle change. But here's the thing—that fear doesn't have to stop you from reaching your sobriety goals. In fact, you can look right in its face and smile, saying, "Yes, I've never been more sure in my life."

So, how do we transform the paralysis of fear into the action of change? First, you have to recognize that fear isn't just an enemy. It's also a teacher, and it points directly to the things that matter most. In other words, if you ask yourself why you're afraid of quitting, you'll discover what you actually find to be the most important. A fear of losing friends due to sobriety shows you that you value social connections, while a fear of failure shows that you care about success. When you take the time to understand what your fears are trying to tell you, you can start to address them constructively.

Building resilience is another vital piece of the puzzle. Resilience is your mental fortitude, an attribute you can develop through deliberate practice. A valuable technique to foster this is something I've called "scenario spinning." When you fear the worst-case scenarios—like facing a party sober—challenge yourself to rewrite the situation into terms that give you control or change how you view the scenario. For example, what if you redefine what a party means to you? It's no longer synonymous with drinking but with celebrating life, connecting with friends, and creating memorable moments. Initially, the thought of attending a party sober might fill you with dread, but reimagining these events from a place of sobriety can reveal their true essence. Scenario spinning can help turn even the most frightening aspects of sobriety into something more manageable.

Maintaining sobriety hinges on motivation. You have to motivate yourself in order to consistently reach your goals, and those goals have to be based on your visions and dreams —as well as based on reality. Being kind to yourself by offering yourself actionable goals is vital. Moreover, understanding and leveraging your fears, strengthening your resilience, and embracing change are your guides along this journey. As we move into the next chapter, we'll build on these foundations, exploring specific strategies for laying the groundwork for sobriety and thriving in your new alcohol-free reality. The journey continues, and trust me, it's worth every step.

STEP #4

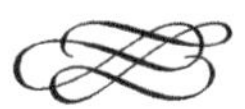

LAYING THE GROUNDWORK FOR SOBRIETY

If you were going to build a house, you wouldn't simply pile bricks haphazardly, anticipating that they would form a sturdy structure. Instead, you'd start with a strong foundation, selecting the most appropriate materials and assembling them into a reliable team. The path to sobriety is kind of like this process, where in order for your "house" to come to life, you have to start with a strong foundation. But instead of bricks, we're talking about a foundation of supportive people, strategies, and more to help you along your journey. Let's find out what it takes to achieve this.

CREATING A SUPPORT SYSTEM: FINDING ALLIES IN YOUR JOURNEY

Recovery is something you can do alone, but like building that house we were talking about, it becomes much easier when you have a team of supporters lending a helping hand. When it comes to sobriety, your journey will be much more effective if you identify your allies and people who can support you. You don't have to brave sobriety alone, and in fact, a support system eases the hardships you will face.

Identifying Supportive People

First and foremost, let's delve into the essence of your support circle. These individuals will be your anchors through tricky times and your biggest cheerleaders during triumphs. Identifying these key players involves evaluating who in your life uplifts you rather than depletes your energy. Especially for those accustomed to prioritizing others' needs over their own, now is the moment to invert that dynamic, allowing others to support your needs instead.

Whether the people you trust to support you are relatives, friends, or co-workers, their pivotal role is to consistently provide you with positive support and sincere care. Take time now to identify these people and reflect on who genuinely supports you and who actively encourages your progress. This is the first step in finding out who is a true part of your support network.

Engaging With Support Groups

Having supportive friends and family is crucial, but not everyone is fortunate enough to have such people to lean on. Whether that's your situation or you're just looking to boost your network, there's an added layer of understanding and empathy found within support groups. These groups, such as Alcoholics Anonymous or SMART Recovery, create a sense of belonging with others who genuinely understand the journey you're on. People in such groups can also contribute to your recovery by offering perspectives and support that those who have never faced addiction might not be able to give.

My path of seeking support from support groups began with the anonymity of online Zoom calls, as the thought of face-to-face meetings was terrifying. However, as my confidence grew, so did my willingness to engage in person. It's important to remember that each journey to sobriety is unique, and what serves one person well may not suit another. So, don't be afraid to personalize your journey and find what works best for you. In these groups, you're embraced by a wealth of shared wisdom, experiences, and encouragement, and you truly don't have anything to be afraid of—even if fear looms strong at first.

Setting Boundaries With Non-Supportive People

Not everyone will be eager to support your journey toward sobriety, and that's perfectly okay. People don't have to support you, and encountering skepticism, criticism, or outright resistance is not uncommon. Rather than focusing on people who don't support you and trying to mold your recovery to their needs, it's important to set healthy boundaries that put yourself first. Establishing boundaries doesn't mean that you have to isolate yourself from others. Instead, it means defining what behaviors you find acceptable and what behaviors you don't, ensuring your interactions remain positive and supportive.

Through my own experiences, I learned that interactions while under the influence were neither productive nor meaningful as I tried to recover. This revelation led me to establish clear boundaries, even with those closest to me. While some relationships may not withstand this transition, remember that more supportive, understanding connections will emerge as you find people who *do* support you. I had friends leave and friends stay, and those friends who left made room for new, more supportive friends to join my circle. Setting boundaries is an act of self-care and a fundamental step in safeguarding your sobriety.

The Role of Accountability

Think about having a workout buddy. On days that you'd rather stay in bed, knowing someone is waiting for you can be the nudge you need to get moving. The same goes for sobriety. Having an accountability partner—a friend, family member, or someone from your support group—can significantly enhance your chances of sustaining sobriety. This person can help keep you on track, remind you of your goals, and be a sounding board when you face challenges. Sometimes, knowing someone is rooting for you and holding you accountable is enough to steer you away from temptation. You can ask someone to be your accountability partner—be it someone in real life or online—and let them know what you need from them as they fill that role.

Reflect and Engage

Grab that list of supportive people you thought of earlier. Next to each name, jot down one specific thing they can help you with on your sobriety journey. It could be a weekly check-in call, joining you for a walk, or simply sending a daily encouraging text. Then, take the bold step of reaching out to them, sharing your goals, and asking if they'd be willing to support you in that specific way. Actively engaging your support network strengthens your resources and reaffirms your commitment to sobriety.

THE SOBRIETY BLUEPRINT: PLANNING YOUR PATH TO RECOVERY

The next thing we have to do is craft your sobriety plan. Crafting your sobriety plan is like drawing out a treasure map for your journey. It includes the routes you'll take, the challenges you'll dodge, and the tools you'll use to find that treasure, which, in this case, is a successful and sober life. This plan is your blueprint—tailored to fit your life's architecture and address the specific nooks and crannies where alcohol used to hide.

Creating a Personalized Plan

First up, let's sketch out your plan. Every good blueprint starts with an understanding of the landscape. Reflect on what your drinking habits looked like. What times of day were you most likely to drink? What activities or emotions triggered your drinking? Answers to these questions will guide the structure of your plan. For instance, if you find that stress from work leads you to drink in the evenings, part of your plan might involve stress management techniques right after work, like a workout session, painting, or another hobby that soothes you. Or if loneliness triggers your drinking, you might schedule evening calls with a friend or family member or plan to attend social gatherings that align with your interests but are alcohol-free. The goal here is to craft a strategy that proactively fills the gaps where alcohol used to be with activities that enrich rather than drain you.

Next is setting realistic and specific goals, like being sober for the next 24 hours, then a week, and gradually increasing your target. We talked about this earlier when discussing moderation. Each goal should be paired with actionable steps. For instance, "To achieve one week of sobriety, I will attend three AA or other support meetings, schedule two dinners with supportive friends, and spend one hour each evening on my guitar." This method sets a clear path and breaks down the overwhelming concept of "forever sobriety" into manageable pieces.

Anticipating and Planning for Triggers

When it comes to any psychological concern like addiction, something that you have to be mindful of is triggers. A trigger is a form of stimulus that launches your brain into an unwanted, hard-to-control frenzy. You might feel compelled to act on an impulse or feel a certain way, which makes it hard to avoid unwanted habits. Practically speaking, you might feel triggered by bars if you drink at bars often, as I did. Going to a bar might make you feel unable to resist drinking, which means that the bar is a trigger for you.

Understanding your triggers is an important part of being able to lay down the foundation for an unbreakable recovery process. By identifying what triggers you, you're better equipped to avoid potential pitfalls. You can begin by cataloging your triggers and then outline a proactive strategy alongside each. Anything that makes you feel compelled to drink—or makes you feel an emotion that would compel you to drink—is a trigger. For me, the anniversaries of loved ones who have passed away were significant triggers. To navigate these moments, I planned evenings filled with reflection, focusing on gratitude for the peace they've found and the pride they would feel in my journey toward sobriety. Rather than succumbing to the urge to drink, I chose to immerse myself in cherished memories and photographs as a positive replacement for alcohol addiction.

In situations where social pressures might act as triggers, it's wise to have an exit strategy ready—knowing how to refuse a drink or excuse yourself gracefully—should the environment become too challenging. Similarly, when specific emotions threaten to derail your sobriety, having a set of immediate, alternative activities can be incredibly beneficial. This might involve plans like engaging in a brisk workout, reaching out to a supportive friend, or dedicating time to a focus-intensive hobby like model building or knitting. These preemptive measures effectively shift the control from your triggers back into your hands.

Emergency Plan for Cravings

Cravings can strike like sudden storms; an emergency plan is your umbrella. This might include a list of reasons you want to stay sober—something you can pull out of your purse or wallet and read to remind yourself why you started this path. Include a few key contacts you can call to talk down a craving, like a friend or support group member. Also, keep some physical tools handy: stress balls, puzzle books, or a sketch pad—anything that keeps your hands and mind busy until the craving passes. Personally, I decided to create a playlist of songs that motivated or calmed me, which helped me to combat the urge to drink.

As you implement these strategies, I want to remind you that the effectiveness of your sobriety blueprint lies in your hands. It should be designed uniquely for you, flexible enough to adjust as you grow, and sturdy enough to support you as you build a life of sobriety. Each day you follow this blueprint, you reinforce the foundation of your sober life, brick by brick, until one day, you look back and see just how far you've come.

HEALTHY SUBSTITUTES FOR ALCOHOL: MANAGING CRAVINGS WITH BETTER CHOICES

Sometimes, the urge to reach for a drink feels like an old friend calling your name from the back of your mind. It's familiar, it's easy, and it's there. But what if you redirected that energy into something that distracts you and enriches your life instead of answering that old call? Let's explore some creative, fulfilling, and healthy alternatives to alcohol that can satisfy your need for a healthy ritual.

To start, think about what role alcohol used to fill for you. There are many different holes in life that people try to fill with alcohol. People use it as a

- way to unwind from a stressful day
- method to socialize with people using alcohol as a shared interest

- quick way to escape from the daily stressors they face
- technique for avoidance or self-medication, even for "innocent" purposes like sleep

Understanding the specific reasons you turned to alcohol in the first place can guide you toward healthier alternatives that fulfill those exact needs. For example, for unwinding, consider a nightly tea ritual. The kettle's gentle whistle, the aromatic steam rising from your cup, and the warm, calming sensation with each sip all contribute to your ability to relax even more effectively than what alcohol used to offer. Herbal teas like chamomile or peppermint are soothing and offer health benefits, from aiding digestion to improving sleep (Rios, 2023).

If socializing was your primary association with drinking, you can pivot to fun activities and keep your hands and mind engaged. Think about game nights—board games, card games, or interactive video games. These settings can be incredibly social and high-spirited without a drop of alcohol. They require focus and teamwork, providing a natural high from the joy of play and the laughter of good company. Plus, winning that game of strategy or teamwork can give you a sense of achievement and connection that alcohol never could. And if you need something tasty to sip on, you can't go wrong with juice, soda, and sparkling waters at these events.

If you're prone to turning to alcohol as a means of stress relief, consider the empowerment of physical activity. Exercise is renowned for its ability to release endorphins, which we talked about earlier. Options are plentiful and can suit any preference or lifestyle. You don't have to hit the gym if you don't want to—a yoga mat or walking around your neighborhood can be just as meaningful if you engage with those forms of exercise regularly. These activities offer a wholesome alternative to alcohol for stress relief and reinforce your dedication to sobriety.

Revitalizing Your Nutrition

Shifting gears a bit, let's talk about nutrition. It's no secret that alcohol can deplete your body of essential nutrients, so part of your recovery involves nourishing your body back to health. This means engaging with targeted nutrition that supports your recovery and reduces cravings. Foods rich in amino acids, like turkey, cottage cheese, and nuts, can boost serotonin levels, improving your mood and reducing the urge to reach for a drink (Sissons, 2018). Opting for the complex carbohydrates in whole grains, fruits, and vegetables can help stabilize your blood sugar by preventing spikes and curbing the mood swings that can lead to cravings (*Get to Know Carbs | ADA*, n.d.). And let's not forget omega-3 fatty acids in fish like salmon and sardines, which can improve brain function and mental health, making it easier to stay on track with your sobriety (Hjalmarsdottir, 2018).

Incorporating these foods into your diet is more than mere nourishment; it becomes an integral part of your recovery journey where food is used as medicine, healing the damage done and paving the way to better health. Each meal presents an opportunity to affirm your health and dedication to sobriety. You can even think of meal preparation as a new ritual that replaces the act of drinking. This process invites you to engage deeply with the ingredients and the act of cooking, finding joy and satisfaction in creating something that nourishes both body and soul. To support this process, I prioritize avoiding processed foods, recognizing that their long shelf life, indicated by extended expiration dates, often signifies a high content of preservatives. In all, mindful approaches to eating underscores the commitment to a healthier, sober lifestyle.

Mindfulness for Cravings Management

Now, let's dig deeper into mindfulness and its role in managing cravings. Mindfulness is a technique that involves being present in the moment, fully aware of your thoughts and feelings without judgment (MINDFUL STAFF, 2020). When a craving hits, instead of automatically reacting to it, mindfulness teaches you to pause, observe the craving for what it is—an urge that will pass—and choose how to respond.

Techniques like focused breathing, where you concentrate solely on your breath, can help center your thoughts and calm your mind, reducing the intensity of the craving. You can also try a body scan, where you move your attention gradually through different body parts and remain mindful of how each part of your body feels. This can help connect you to the physical reality of the moment, distancing you from the craving. Mindfulness can also be applied through mindful eating, where you eat slowly, savoring each bite and genuinely experiencing the flavors, textures, and smells of your meal. This practice makes eating more enjoyable and can lead to better digestion and satisfaction with smaller portions, which is essential when you're replacing a habit that involves consuming a substance mindlessly.

Incorporating these mindfulness techniques into your daily routine can change how you experience cravings and what you do to manage them. They teach you to live in the present and appreciate the now, giving you the tools to manage your life and recovery with intention and grace. Rather than caving in the face of a craving, mindfulness allows you to focus on what you can control in a healthy, regulated way. Each mindful moment is a step away from past habits and a step toward a balanced, sober life where cravings have less power and you have more.

THE ROLE OF PROFESSIONAL HELP: WHEN TO SEEK COUNSELING OR THERAPY

Sometimes, the path to sobriety feels like you're trying to assemble furniture without the instruction manual—frustrating and more complicated than it needs to be. That's where professional help comes into play. Professionals like therapists, counselors, and psychiatrists can help you out by working with you to find the instruction manual that matches your needs and offering tools along the way. Recognizing when you might need to reach out for this kind of help is crucial on your road to recovery.

So, when is it time to seek professional support? Consider this step if you find yourself swamped by emotions, if your emotional state is as unpredictable as a rollercoaster, or if, no matter how hard you try, maintaining sobriety feels like an elusive goal. It's particularly important if you're grappling with underlying mental health issues such as depression, anxiety, or unresolved trauma, which often lurk in the shadows, undermining your journey to sobriety. Professional therapists or doctors are skilled at navigating these intricate challenges, and they can offer a confidential environment to delve into your feelings, understand your behaviors and urges, and forge strategies for living a fulfilling life without alcohol dependency.

My journey with professional support was incredibly beneficial; my doctor was readily available for online consultations, which meant that we could adjust my treatment plan and medications as needed. When it came to counseling, I initially reached out daily with just a short text or by reading about my past accomplishments. Professional help can look like whatever you need it to look like along your journey, so don't feel like you have to stick to some rigid constraints for it.

If you're interested in professional help, it can be good to know about the different types of therapeutic approaches commonly used to treat alcohol addiction. There are a few different approaches you might find available to you (Murray, 2020):

- **Cognitive Behavioral Therapy (CBT)**: CBT is a method of therapy that involves pointing out your negative thoughts and replacing them with positive thoughts and behaviors. This is super helpful for cravings because it shifts a tendency to drink to a tendency to engage with positive, constructive behaviors. This includes challenging negative

thoughts, managing fears, and developing skills to support healthy coping.
- **Motivational Interviewing**: Motivational interviewing can help if you're struggling to identify your motivations for sobriety. If you feel powerless or like you don't really care, then motivational interviewing is an incredible option for you.
- **Dialectical Behavioral Therapy (DBT)**: DBT is similar to CBT, but it assumes that everything you think, do, and feel is related. From this belief, DBT works to provide you with skills that help you find emotional balance and regulate your emotions through distress tolerance, social skills, and mindfulness.

You can start by seeking the method that speaks to you the most or trying out a combination of methods. It might take several attempts to find someone whose expertise and approach genuinely resonate with you. You can begin your search by asking for recommendations from your primary care physician or members of local support groups. During initial consultations with potential therapists, make sure to discuss your specific goals and verify their familiarity with issues related to alcohol dependency. This will help you discover whether you feel with a particular professional. If the connection with the first therapist doesn't feel right, don't give up—your ideal match exists and might take a few tries to find.

As we close this chapter on laying the groundwork for sobriety, remember that building a solid foundation involves understanding yourself deeply, crafting a personal and proactive plan, and sometimes, leaning on professional expertise. Each step you take, supported by friends, routines, or counselors, is a step toward sobriety and a fuller, more prosperous life beyond alcohol. Next, we'll explore more in-depth tips and tricks for really shedding the skin of alcohol addiction.

STEP #5

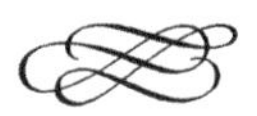

IDENTIFYING KEY STRATEGIES FOR QUITTING ALCOHOL

By now, we've gained a ton of skills to help you on your journey. From understanding the value of social and professional support to navigating healthy habits and more, you have tools in your arsenal that can help you fight against addiction. Now, it's time for the next level when it comes to strategies for quitting. In this chapter, we're going to spend ample time dissecting the pros and cons, navigating the twists and turns, and discovering how to choose the right path for you. Buckle up; it's going to be an insightful ride!

GOING COLD TURKEY VS. GRADUAL REDUCTION: PROS AND CONS

In the first days of my journey, I asked myself a big question: Should I stop drinking completely or take it little by little? For some people, quitting cold turkey is the way to go; for others, this approach can be relapse-inducing, if not outright dangerous. Determining which path is for you is going to take some careful consideration of a few different things.

Immediate vs. Gradual

When you quit drinking cold turkey, it's like jumping directly into the deep end. It's abrupt, tough, and boy, does it test your spirit? You stop all alcohol at once, and the change to your body and brain is immediate and often intense. The advantage here? You're essentially ripping off the Band-Aid of sobriety. You face the withdrawal head-on, and for some, the idea of getting through the worst of it quickly is appealing. It's a clean break, with no ambiguity about limits or slipping back into old habits, and for some people, this can make the journey far easier.

On the flip side, you have the gradual reduction route. This is like slowly easing into colder waters, letting your body adjust bit by bit. You reduce your alcohol consumption over time, which can be less of a shock to your system, both physically and mentally. This method can feel more manageable if you feel like you may be intimidated by the severity of immediate withdrawal or if you have health concerns that make sudden withdrawal riskier. It allows you to maintain a semblance of normalcy as you slowly remove alcohol from your life as well, which can be less disruptive to your daily functioning.

Physical Health Impacts

When you quit cold turkey, your body, used to having a certain level of alcohol regularly, might react a bit dramatically, especially if you've been a long-time drinker. We talked about the withdrawal symptoms earlier, and the physical ones are often immediate and hard to manage. Your nervous system has to recalibrate, and this process can be rough. However, this can be more manageable for those who would rather suffer intensely for two or three days and be done with it than suffer bit by bit for weeks.

In contrast, gradual reduction, by its nature, might mitigate some of these intense reactions, but it also extends the time when you feel moderately unwell. By slowly dialing down your alcohol intake, you give your body a chance to adjust to lower levels of alcohol over time, which can help ease the severity of withdrawal symptoms. However, this method requires careful monitoring and control, and maintaining control when it comes to drinking isn't always easy for everyone.

Psychological Readiness

Your level of psychological readiness is important to think of, too. Mentally, going cold turkey requires a significant amount of willpower and readiness. If you're planning to go cold turkey, it's best to be prepared for the emotional and psychological fallout that can accompany that choice.

Gradual reduction, meanwhile, can be less daunting psychologically. It allows for a more measured approach to facing life without alcohol, which can be less of a shock to your system and your lifestyle. It also gives you time to develop new coping mechanisms as you decrease your alcohol intake, rather than having to overhaul your coping strategies all at once.

Success Rates and Personal Fit

Here's where it gets personal. Success rates for either method vary widely or depend on your unique situation. It is important to remember that everyone is different. In some cases, for those with severe addiction, medically supervised cold turkey might be necessary. For others, especially those who might not have access to immediate professional support, a gradual reduction could offer a more achievable path to sobriety.

The key is to honestly assess not just your drinking habits but also your support system, your health, and your personal history of addiction. No two people are the same, and no one method fits all. Maybe you need the immediacy of cold turkey to commit to change, or perhaps you find reassurance in the more forgiving pace of gradual reduction. Remember, the best method is the one that you realistically can stick to, that keeps you safe and ultimately leads you to a healthier, sober life.

Reflect and Choose

Consider this as you ponder your path: Which method aligns with your lifestyle, responsibilities, and health? Try writing out a pros and cons list for each method, reflecting on past attempts to quit, your daily routine, and how each technique might fit into your life. This can help you choose the strategy that best fits your life, setting yourself up for sobriety and success.

NAVIGATING WITHDRAWAL: PRACTICAL TIPS AND MEDICAL INSIGHTS

Withdrawal is like being the main character in a horror movie—sweaty, shaky, and unsure when the next jump scare of craving will hit. But the thing is, you can be the hero in this flick if you come armed with the right strategies and a crew of supporters. This means knowing how to manage those pesky withdrawal symptoms. For example, the first line of defense? Good old H2O—water. Staying hydrated is important during withdrawal and can help mitigate some symptoms—like headaches and nausea—that you might experience. It also helps flush out the toxins from drinking, which can speed the early stages of withdrawal up (Pinelands Recovery Center Staff, 2022).

There's also food to think about. During withdrawal, your body is doing some heavy lifting, trying to repair itself from the inside out, and it needs the right kind of nutrients to do so. Lean proteins, fruits, and veggies are your best friends here. These foods are nutrient-rich and can, therefore, help repair damage caused by alcohol (Bridges of Hope, 2023). Foods rich in amino acids and complex carbohydrates, as discussed earlier, can help reboot your neurotransmitter production and stabilize mood, which is crucial as well.

But what if things get too intense? What if hydration and nutrition aren't enough to keep the withdrawal beasts at bay? This is where professional detox programs come into play. Programs like this might seem scary, but they're a really great way to ensure your health and safety as you recover. They provide medical supervision, which can be helpful because withdrawal can sometimes swing from "kind of uncomfortable" to a "scary medical emergency" pretty quickly. Medications can be used to safely manage symptoms like seizures or severe anxiety in these programs, making the detox process smoother and safer without leading to a second addiction.

On the emotional front, withdrawal can feel messy, confusing, and sometimes straight-up overwhelming. That's why it's important to identify those supportive people—friends, family, or your support group—who can be there for you. Emotional support during this phase isn't just lovely; it's essential. Having people around who can remind you why you started this path when you're knee-deep in withdrawal muck is inspiring, motivating, and important in moments where recovery seems harder than anything. Just knowing you're not alone in this can be incredibly helpful.

Withdrawal is challenging, but with a mix of self-care strategies, professional help, and a support network, you've got a fighting chance—no, a guarantee—to come out on the other side, surviving *and* thriving. As you gear up to face this challenge, remember that each symptom managed, each craving resisted, and each day completed is a victory. It's you, turning the page, ready to start a new chapter in your life where you're in control.

LEVERAGING MINDFULNESS AND MEDITATION IN YOUR SOBRIETY JOURNEY

Let's chat about mindfulness, shall we? I mean, we've talked about it a little bit already, but we haven't really sat and taken the time to fully piece it into recovery as a strategy. Mindfulness is a skill that allows you to tune into the present moment with full attention without letting past regrets or future anxieties take the wheel. The beauty of mindfulness in managing stress and cravings is that it teaches you to observe these feelings without judgment and without feeling like you have to take immediate action to "solve" those feelings. Through mindfulness, you learn to recognize your thoughts and feelings as passing clouds in a vast sky—visible but not defining the whole sky.

One way that you can implement mindfulness as a part of your recovery is through the world of daily meditation practices. Meditation isn't what people often think of it as. You don't have to do it sitting cross-legged surrounded by candles (unless that's your vibe, of course!). It can be as simple as spending five minutes each morning focusing on your breath. For example, try this exercise:

1. Find a quiet spot and sit comfortably.
2. Close your eyes, take a deep breath for 5 seconds, hold it for 5 seconds, and exhale slowly for 5 seconds.
3. Focus on the sensation of air filling your lungs and leaving your body.
4. If your mind wanders to your to-do list or what's for dinner, gently bring it back to your breath.

This practice allows you to find a space of relaxation while building your focus and calming your mind, making you less reactive to the cravings or stress that might have led you to drink before.

Also, it helps if you adopt a mindset of neutrality, not judgment. Next time a craving hits, you can pause and observe it with curiosity instead of wrestling with it. Where do you feel it in your body? Could you share any thoughts about it? By observing it, you're stepping back and reducing its power over you. Then, use your breath as an anchor—focus on each inhale and exhale until the craving loses its urgency. You don't have to force the craving away; managing it with grace and without automatically reaching for alcohol is an amazing start.

Building a mindful lifestyle supports long-term sobriety and overall well-being by infusing your daily life with practices that enhance awareness and self-control. Start small. You can begin by practicing mindful eating, where you pay attention to your food's taste, texture, and enjoyment rather than eating mechanically. If that's not your thing, you can try mindful walking—where you focus on the sensation of your feet touching the ground, the sounds around you, and the feeling of the air on your skin. Each mindful practice that you integrate into your life strengthens your ability to stay present and engaged, reducing the need to escape into old habits like drinking.

Integrating mindfulness into your life doesn't mean you need to become a Zen master or spend hours meditating each day. It just means taking strides to experience your life more fully as it happens and being awake rather than numb or distracted. This awakening makes life richer, makes colors brighter, and strengthens your ability to deal with challenges.

THE IMPORTANCE OF ROUTINE: STRUCTURING YOUR DAY WITHOUT ALCOHOL

When you remove a habit, it leaves a gap in your life, and that gap is a place for opportunity. When you stop drinking, the gap left by that habit can be used to improve your life, or it can be used to make a negative impact. This is where creating a sober routine comes into play, filling that gap in your day with stable, supportive routines and actions that keep your day moving smoothly from one activity to the next.

Building a daily routine that supports your sobriety goes beyond just cutting alcohol out; it also involves intentionally structuring your day to foster stability and minimize stress, which can be a trigger for relapse, by adding positive habits in. You can start creating these positive routines by thinking about the natural rhythm of your day. When are you most energetic? When do you feel most vulnerable? You can use your understanding of your daily rhythms to tailor your routine in such a way that enhances your strengths and protects your weak points. For example, if mornings are tough, start your day with an activity that sets a positive tone, like a walk, a good breakfast, or a few minutes of meditation. This creates a positive domino effect, making it easier to maintain your sobriety throughout the day.

Incorporate work, leisure, and self-care in balanced measures, too. Too much idle time can be dangerous when you're used to filling it with drinking. Structure your work hours if you're working, and pencil in regular breaks to avoid burnout and stress that can trigger a post-work craving. For leisure, choose activities that engage you and bring you joy without involving alcohol. It could be anything from reading to rock climbing. Don't skimp on self-care; ensure you have time for adequate sleep, nutrition, and relaxation. Taking care of yourself isn't a luxury; it's an essential that keeps your positive habits and progress aligned without toppling over into the danger zone of a relapse.

The role of structure in recovery cannot be overstated. A well-planned day reduces the chaos that can lead to anxiety and uncertainty—emotions that might have previously driven you to drink. Having a clear outline of what your day holds eliminates much of the guesswork and reduces the risk of being caught off-guard by triggers. This doesn't mean your schedule has to be rigid or military-like; rather, having a predictable framework within which flexibility can exist helps you feel solace in those healthy routines. This predictable pattern can significantly ease anxiety, as you know what to expect and what you're moving toward.

Adapting your routine over time is also important as your recovery evolves and your needs change. What works in the early days of your sobriety might be less effective six months later, which is why you should stay flexible and responsive to your growth. Maybe you've discovered a new passion for which you want to make more time, or you've realized you need more downtime as your work responsibilities increase. Regularly revisiting and revising your routine to fit in these observations and maintain fulfillment is critical. It ensures that your daily structure effectively supports your sobriety, adapts as you do, and always aligns with your current needs and goals.

FINDING JOY IN SOBER ACTIVITIES: REPLACING OLD HABITS WITH NEW PASSIONS

Remember when social gatherings or winding down meant reaching for a drink? It was easy, almost automatic. Imagine filling that part of your life, that "glass," with something else that doesn't give you a hangover or regrets. Let's talk about rediscovering joy in activities, not around alcohol. This means rekindling old passions or discovering new interests that enrich your life and support your sobriety.

Passionate Activities and Exploration

When was the last time you did something just for the fun of it, not because it was a default option at a social event? At one point in my life, the only answer that I had to this question was, "I don't know." A whole world of interests and hobbies awaits, and they don't involve alcohol. From painting and writing to hiking and coding, these activities can be more than simply time-fillers; they can be the door that opens to new joys and circles of like-minded friends.

You can start discovering new hobbies or dipping into activities you might enjoy by listing things you have always wanted to try but have yet to do. Maybe you were interested in photography or fancied trying your hand at pottery. Why not now? Sobriety means that you have hours upon hours to try new things when previously you spent that time drinking. It means that you have the energy and vitality to support those activities, too. Moreover, learning something new can be incredibly rewarding and a powerful distraction from any cravings you might experience.

The benefits of engaging in sober hobbies are plentiful. They improve your mental and physical health, giving you something tangible to show for your time (like a photograph, a piece of art, or a healthier body from physical activities). These hobbies boost your mood and self-esteem, providing a sense of accomplishment that no glass of wine or beer can match. Plus, the focus required for most hobbies can act as a form of meditation, helping you stay present and mindful, all while reducing stress without needing to numb it with alcohol.

Sober Socializing

Socializing without alcohol might seem daunting at first. It might feel like you're the only one not holding a drink at parties or gatherings. In these moments, something you have to remember is that you're not alone. Many people are choosing to reduce their alcohol intake or abstain altogether, and they're having a great time doing it. You can join the club by exploring social activities that aren't centered around drinking. Join a sports league, take a group class at a local community center, or volunteer. These activities can offer new ways to connect with people and build friendships based on shared interests rather than drinks.

If you do want to go out and enjoy your time while other people are drinking, you also have a few options. Knowing what you're going to say can help reduce anxiety while still allowing you to enjoy a night out. My favorite line when I went out with friends who asked if I wanted a drink was, "Sure, I'll have a Sprite!" This asserted that "a drink" doesn't have to be alcohol, all while making sure I didn't feel like the odd one out for saying no outright. You can also just say, "No, I'm not drinking," or even, "I don't drink anymore," if you're comfortable sharing. It also helps to have a go-to alcohol-free drink that you enjoy and can order at dinner when it might feel uncomfortable to have an empty spot at the table in front of you. And hey, *water* is a good choice no matter who you are!

Quitting alcohol can be tricky, especially when you have to ask yourself questions like, "Cold turkey or gradual?" and, "What am I going to do with my time instead?" However, with the strategies for quitting provided to you in this chapter, your journey to recovery has been leveled up. Next, we'll take a look at how to maintain the progress you're making and ensure that your sober life grows and enriches you despite some of the common hurdles recovering alcohol addicts face. Stay tuned and remember: each day is a new opportunity to add color and joy to your sober canvas. Let's keep painting a masterpiece.

The Turning Point

Believe you can, and you're halfway there.

— THEODORE ROOSEVELT

What was the moment that you realized you needed to take action? Can you pinpoint it? For me, it was that trip to the doctor that confirmed everything I feared... but I knew before that. That's why I went to the doctor in the first place. Maybe part of me hoped that nothing would show up on the bloodwork, and I'd be able to carry on as I had been... and maybe part of me hoped that it would, and I would be forced to get the help I needed.

If you're familiar with that "I don't care. Have another drink" mentality that I used to lean on, then your narrative might be similar: If you don't care, it means you *know*, and part of what that next drink is doing is helping you hide it from yourself. Usually what happens then is a specific event that shows you it's time to do something about your addiction. For me, it was the blood test. For someone else, it might be a mistake that could have been avoided if they hadn't been drinking – most likely a harmful one. Whatever that moment is, it's significant... and it's something each of us goes through.

While you're thinking about that moment and the pain you associate with it, I'd like to call on your empathy for other people who've experienced a similar turning point, and ask you to share this information with them. That sounds like a big ask when you're already dealing with so much, but it's a lot easier than you think – all you need to do is leave a short review.

By leaving a review of this book on Amazon, you'll show those who are looking for this help exactly where they can find it.

Your review will contribute to new readers spending less time searching for help and connecting more quickly with the guidance they're looking for. I don't have to tell you how powerful reviews are for helping people select the books that are right for them, and seeing the opinions of other people who are in the same boat is so valuable.

Thank you so much for your support. This journey isn't an easy one; we need all the help we can get.

Scan the QR code below

Or Put this link into your browser

https://www.amazon.com/review/review-your-purchases/?asin=B0D9CCTL7Z

STEP #6

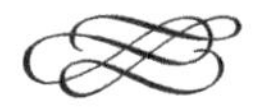

OVERCOMING COMMON HURDLES

You're at a friend's wedding, surrounded by the clinks of glasses and the merry chatter of celebration. There's laughter, dancing, and your well-meaning friend heading your way with a champagne flute just for you. It's like being a kid in a dodgeball game, and you've just been handed the ball. What do you do? Toss it back politely, or find a clever way to dodge it? This chapter is all about navigating those tricky situations where alcohol swings back into your spotlight in any form, not with temptation but as a curveball that you need to catch and throw back with confidence. Trust me, I was once terrified at the mere prospect of facing situations like these, but with the tips and tricks in this chapter, common hurdles were no match for me.

HANDLING SOCIAL PRESSURE: SAYING NO WITH CONFIDENCE

One of the many challenges you'll face as a recovering alcohol addict is social pressure. There are dozens of places and events where drinking is treated the same as showing up —you're there, or you're not—and knowing how to show up without having to sober up the next day is key.

Tip #1: Be Assertive

Assertiveness doesn't mean being forceful or mean; instead, it means deciding what roles alcohol plays in your life and making sure that no one impedes your right to make that decision. Saying no to a drink can feel like you're turning down more than just a beverage—you might worry it seems you're rejecting someone's kindness or company. But here, let's reshape that script. Assertiveness is really about expressing your needs and boundaries respectfully and clearly. Practice simple, straightforward responses like, "Thanks, but I'm not drinking tonight" or "I'm keeping it clear-headed today!" Deliver it with a smile. It's not a defense; it's a declaration of your choices. If you're met with pushback, keep your cool. Repeat your stance, and remember that a good friend is going to be respectful of your choices.

Tip #2: Planning Ahead for Social Events

Before stepping out to any event where alcohol is the guest of honor, have your strategy polished. Decide beforehand what you'll drink instead, as I mentioned earlier. Maybe line up a favorite nonalcoholic beverage, like a soda with lime or a fancy mocktail, so your hands aren't empty, and you're less likely to be offered a drink. Have your "why" ready, too. Sometimes, sharing a bit of your story can turn awkwardness into admiration. People often respect honesty and might even share their own experiences. Lastly, always have an exit strategy. If the event becomes too centered around drinking, and you're feeling uncomfortable, know how you can leave gracefully. I am not shy and a bit of a jokester, so sometimes, around acquaintances who don't know that I have become AF. I will sometimes say, "Let me ask my liver." Pause, and it's a "no thank you."

Above all, remember that "no" is a good enough response and that you can always leave if you're uncomfortable. It's more important to keep your sobriety intact than it is to have one night of "fun" where people don't respect your boundaries.

Tip #3: Stick With Your Supportive Friends

This journey loves company, especially the supportive kind. Lean on your friends who respect and understand your sobriety. They can be your allies in social settings. Please give them a heads-up about your concerns before an event because often, they'll be more than willing to help you navigate the night, whether by sticking by your side when the toasts roll out or by helping steer conversations away from your drinking habits to more comfortable topics.

Tip #4: Know How to Deal With Peer Pressure

Peer pressure can sneak up on you, often masked as banter or persuasion. It might be one friend who insists you can't leave the party without trying their famous spiked punch or another who says you can't *really* celebrate without getting tipsy. You have to stand your ground in situations like these. True friends won't pressure you to compromise your health or values. They'll respect your "no" even if they don't understand it.

If you find yourself repeatedly in situations where you're being pressured or feel unsupported, it might be time to reevaluate those relationships. It's okay to drift from those who don't support your growth. Sobriety might change your social landscape, and that's okay. It's about finding a tribe that fits your sober blueprint, not altering your blueprint to fit the tribe.

Navigating social settings without alcohol can feel like learning to socialize all over again. You may also be like I was and question who I was because I was always "The drunk" life of the party. It turns out most people liked me better sober and funny than sloppy and not as fun. Initially, you might step on a few toes or feel out of rhythm as you learn a new song and dance. But just know that with each event, each gathering, and each confident "no," you'll find your stride.

DEALING WITH CRAVINGS: SHORT-TERM STRATEGIES FOR LONG-TERM SUCCESS

Dealing with cravings can feel like you're dealing with a surprise ambush at every corner. They pop up unannounced, whether triggered by a stressful day at work or even the whiff of a drink at a friend's gathering, and they shake you up before you have a chance to realize what's happening. One strategy that you can use to help navigate this is keeping a craving journal. Scribble down when cravings hit, what's happening around you, and how you feel. Patterns will emerge, and you can analyze those patterns to see what you need to avoid, when you're safest, and what you can do to keep yourself sober in unpredictable situations. Maybe it's always after those marathon meetings at work or during the lonely Sunday evenings.

Another strategy that you can use to manage cravings is the implementation of distraction techniques. Distracting from the cravings means that you aren't as likely to give in. There are many meaningful and purposeful ways that you can distract yourself, like engaging in a hobby that absorbs your full attention. It could be anything from painting models to strumming a guitar, and you don't have to be a pro to do it. The key is immersion. The more involved you are, the less mental bandwidth you have to spare for cravings. Physical exercise is another brilliant detour. Go for a run, or if you're not one for pounding the pavement, a dance class can skyrocket your heart rate and squash those cravings. Yoga, too, can be a double whammy, offering both physical and mental relief, stretching away the tension, and folding in calm. I also found that a class away from the house is best.

Find people in that group who go every day or at a specific time, and let them know you would like to be an accountability partner. You may say you don't have the funds for this, but I used the money that I saved on booze to make this work.

Managing emotions plays a colossal role in navigating the maze of cravings, too. Sometimes, it's not the event itself but the reactions that send us seeking comfort in old habits. For example, you might not be triggered by a bad day at work, but seeing others despair over it, or feeling that despair yourself, can take the place of a trigger. Developing healthy emotional management skills is important to handling these situations. Techniques can vary from deep breathing exercises, which help maintain calm, to writing out what you feel in a journal, transforming overwhelming anxiety into manageable scripts.

Navigating cravings is a dynamic part of maintaining sobriety. It requires awareness, tools, and a good dose of self-compassion. With each craving you pass, you're moving further from alcohol and closer to the version of yourself you're meant to be.

THE PINK CLOUD AND BEYOND: MANAGING EMOTIONAL UPS AND DOWNS

So, you're a few weeks into your sobriety, and suddenly, everything feels surprisingly awesome. You're waking up clear-headed, full of energy, and buzzing with positive vibes. Welcome to what's affectionately known as the "pink cloud" phase (Stonebraker, 2023). It's the honeymoon period of recovery where everything seems shiny and new, and the struggles of your past relationship with alcohol feel like a distant memory. However, like most honeymoons, this phase doesn't last forever, and it's good to be prepared for the pink cloud to disappear.

The pink cloud is a psychological phase encountered by many who embark on the path of sobriety. It is characterized by a temporary burst of euphoria and optimism in the early stages of alcohol abstinence. In this state, life without alcohol seems thrilling, easy, and enlightening. While riding this cloud, the realities of life can seem less daunting, and the challenges of staying sober may not appear as harsh. However, you have to recognize this stage for what it is—a phase. The real test often begins when the cloud dissipates and the gravity of long-term sobriety sets in with its ups and downs. Being prepared for this is key to preventing a relapse.

The key here is to develop and maintain a balanced perspective. When the euphoria wanes, you may find yourself facing the underlying issues that your addiction masked. This shift can lead to feelings of sadness, anxiety, or doubt—emotions that the pink cloud might have temporarily overshadowed. During these times, you should have the toolkit ready. This toolkit should include all of the activities and practices that anchor you—the ones you've learned in this book and on your own journey. Mindfulness exercises, regular physical activity, and engaging with your hobbies are just a few of the ways you can manage the post-pink cloud vibes. They provide stability, bringing you back to a state of equilibrium.

Building long-term emotional stability requires planning, suitable techniques, and continual maintenance. You can start by setting up a routine incorporating time for self-reflection, such as journaling or meditation, which will help you manage the emotional turmoil after the pink cloud fades from recovery's sky. These practices encourage you to process and release emotions healthily rather than bottling them up until they overflow.

Maintaining hope during the tougher periods of recovery can be challenging, especially because every day won't be sunny. Some days will be downright stormy, and that's okay. During these times, lean on your support system—friends, family, or support groups—and your strategies for coping to carry you through to sunnier times. Just as clouds provide rain to nourish the earth, difficult days can offer lessons that nourish your growth. Embrace them. Keep a list of your achievements, no matter how small, and review it regularly to remind yourself how far you've come. Celebrate the milestones, and let each one serve as a beacon of hope, guiding you through the darker days.

Navigating the decline of the pink cloud and the subsequent emotional fluctuations is just another part of learning to thrive in your new reality. Recognizing and embracing the full spectrum of your emotions and understanding that they are all part of the human experience is important to a healthier and emotionally stable recovery. With the right tools and support, you can weather the storms and enjoy the sunshine, all while building a resilient, fulfilling, and sober life.

RELAPSE: UNDERSTANDING, PREVENTING, AND OVERCOMING IT

If you're playing a video game and get zapped by an unexpected boss and bumped back a few levels, it's frustrating, but it doesn't mean you've lost all your skills or can't beat the game. It just means you've hit a snag in your progress, and now you have more insight into how to maneuver past this point next time. This is a lot like experiencing a relapse in your sobriety. It's not a sign of defeat or an indicator that your progress thus far hasn't been important; it's part of the process for many—a hiccup on the road to recovery that, believe it or not, can make you stronger and more prepared for the journey ahead.

Understanding and Preventing Relapses

Relapse can sometimes feel like a dirty word whispered in the shadows of recovery conversations. People talk about relapse like it's the worst thing on Earth, and I was terrified to admit to the hiccups in my journey because of it. But you know what's worse than relapsing? Giving up because you feel like a relapse is the end of the road. Relapse is common, and it's often part of the recovery process. It doesn't erase the days, weeks, or months of sobriety you've achieved. Each of those days you've spent sober is a victory, and relapse is merely a reminder that recovery requires continuous effort. It's important to give yourself grace in moments like these without judgment or guilt. Understanding that relapse can happen can help you and those around you handle it with compassion rather than criticism. This understanding is non-negotiable if you want to recover because the emotional fallout from feeling like you've failed can sometimes be more damaging than the relapse itself.

Preventing relapse starts with vigilance about your triggers. You've likely gotten to know these triggers quite well by now. With that being said, do what you need to do to keep your triggers at bay, and you've already done half of the work of preventing a relapse. Depending on your needs, this might mean attending support meetings, staying connected with your sober friends, and maybe keeping a journal to help you vent frustrations or celebrate successes. These actions create a routine that supports sobriety and reduces the risk of relapse. Also, having a plan for relapses or managing close calls can make all the difference. This plan could involve identifying signs that you're emotionally slipping and having a list of steps to stabilize your situation, like calling a friend, attending an extra meeting, or engaging in a favorite hobby.

Handling a Relapse

Dealing with a relapse, should it occur, involves a healthy dose of kindness—toward yourself. It's easy to beat yourself up and drown in a pool of guilt, but where's the progress in that? No one has ever succeeded in beating themselves up, and in fact, doing so can make the relapse harder to bounce back from. Instead, treat a relapse as a learning opportunity. Analyze what led up to it without judgment. Was it stressful? Were you feeling isolated? Understanding the "why" behind your relapse can help you know what to do next time.

Once you've gained this understanding, recommit to your sobriety. Contact your support network, be open about your slip, and re-engage with your recovery activities to help get back into the habit of recovery. It's not starting over but rather starting fresh with the learning experience of the relapse in your toolkit. The support of people who understand can be incredibly reinforcing during this time. Remember, every attempt at sobriety, regardless of setbacks, contributes to a longer, healthier, alcohol-free life, and you should be proud of yourself for getting back up when relapse knocks you down.

Navigating the concept of relapse with understanding and preparedness can transform it from a feared enemy into a recognized part of the recovery process. Like that tricky boss level in a video game, each playthrough teaches you something new about how to succeed. With the right strategies and support, you can continue to move forward more robustly and equipped than before, ready to continue your adventure in sobriety with renewed vigor and insight.

NAVIGATING RELATIONSHIPS AS YOU CHANGE: COMMUNICATION AND BOUNDARIES

As you embrace sobriety, you'll notice a ripple effect touching every corner of your life, especially your relationships. This is another challenge you have to master as you heal. The dynamics of your relationships will shift, and that's both okay and expected. Sobriety is going to help you see old interactions in a new light, demonstrating which parts of your relationships stemmed from genuine connection and which parts were propped up by shared drinking habits. This shift calls for open, honest communication about your needs and the new boundaries that support your sober lifestyle.

Communication for Sobriety

Communication is like your relationship's immune system—it keeps things healthy and functioning. When you make the decision to choose sobriety, any relationship that you expect to remain healthy—or to improve in health—necessitates an honest expression of how your needs have evolved since choosing sobriety. This can include discussing how you might no longer attend certain events or explaining why you might leave a gathering early. Doing this helps ensure that your loved ones understand the changes in your behavior and makes sure that they know that those changes aren't personal rejections. Open dialogue can mitigate misunderstandings and foster a supportive environment, and that includes being willing to answer questions and what-ifs that people may have when it comes to your relationship with them.

Setting Your Social Boundaries

Setting healthy boundaries is equally vital. As I mentioned earlier, boundaries aren't walls to keep people out; they are guidelines that help others understand how to respect and support your new lifestyle. For instance, asking friends not to bring alcohol when they come to your house or choosing not to attend events known primarily for drinking is a boundary that you have the right to set. This could change with time, but at the beginning, stay clear of drinks at your AF home.

It's important to communicate these boundaries clearly and assertively, though, because it's not going to be clear what your boundaries are if you never talk about them. At the same time, your communication can't be littered with apologies or framing those boundaries as a negotiable request. Imagine if you were allergic to peanuts—you wouldn't shy away from telling everyone to keep peanuts out of your dishes to make them feel more comfortable. Treat your sobriety with the same level of importance.

Knowing When to Let Go

Not all relationships are going to align with your new sober path, and that's a tough pill to swallow. You might find that some friends, perhaps those with whom you primarily shared drinking experiences, may drift away or even resist your changes. They might try to convince you to have "just one drink" or stop inviting you to gatherings. It's painful, but it's also a part of growth. Let yourself be okay with distancing yourself from relationships that threaten your sobriety or no longer contribute positively to your life. It doesn't mean you care about these people any less; you're simply prioritizing your health and well-being. I let go of several "Drinking buddies", they were not true friends.

At the same time, your recovery and newfound mindset toward socialization is a golden opportunity to strengthen relationships with those who support you and your sobriety. Invest time and energy into these relationships, prioritizing them above relationships where people don't seem to support you. With these friends, make it a habit to engage in activities together that don't involve alcohol—go hiking, take a cooking class, or start a joint project. These experiences create new, joyful memories and reinforce the bonds that support your new lifestyle, placing bonding and adventure above any bottle, can, or glass.

Navigating the changing dynamics of relationships as you embrace sobriety is a delicate dance of communication, boundary-setting, and, sometimes, letting go. It involves building a community around you that echoes back the commitment you've made to yourself, offering support and understanding in place of judgment and temptation. As you continue to evolve, so will your relationships. Keep the lines of communication open, hold your boundaries with confidence, and cherish those who walk this path with you. Equally as important is being sure to respect yourself when setbacks come your way and handling relapse with grace and self-compassion. Challenges aren't the end of the road for your recovery.

Remember that each challenge you face on your path, big or small, offers an opportunity for growth. Whether learning to say no with confidence, managing cravings, or navigating the emotional waves of recovery, you are gaining incredible skills that make you stronger. In the next chapter, we'll explore how you can keep strengthening yourself by focusing on your physical well-being through nutrition, exercise, and self-care.

STEP #7

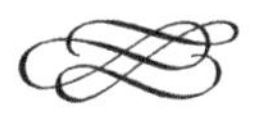

ENHANCING PHYSICAL WELL-BEING

When it comes to getting sober and overcoming addiction, the health benefits focused on most are the ones pertaining to your mind. And don't get me wrong, those mental health benefits are spectacular, but what about the body? And I'm not just talking about the health benefits that you gain from putting down the bottle—I'm also talking about the physical health benefits that you create for yourself through conscious decisions to enhance your physical well-being. Recovery is more than what you gain from stopping a bad habit; it's also what you gain for loving yourself enough to gain new ones, and that includes caring for your body. These are all recommendations and do not come easily for some. For example, I could not give up my 2 cups of coffee a day.

NUTRITION FOR RECOVERY: FOODS THAT HEAL BODY AND MIND

We've talked a little bit about nutrition already—about how you can eat certain things to balance your mood and improve your brain's ability to function. It's time to power up your recovery nutrition knowledge because we're digging deeper.

Balanced Diet Benefits

Let's start with the basics: a balanced diet. Each aspect of a balanced diet—carbohydrates, proteins, fats, vitamins, and minerals—has a specific role in repairing your body and bolstering your brain health. There are some things you should 100% include, and a few you should avoid, for a balanced diet:

- **Carbohydrates**: A lot of people believe that carbs are bad for you, but they aren't. In fact, carbohydrates are your body's primary source of energy, which means that supporting a healthy, energetic lifestyle relies on eating enough healthy carbs (*Carbohydrates*, n.d.).
- **Protein**: Protein-rich foods are like a first-aid kit for the body, helping to repair muscles and damage sustained throughout the day (Wang et al., 2022). They give your body strength, and you can never have too much strength in the face of addiction.
- **Healthy fats**: Healthy fats and fatty acids support functions within the brain, offering improved cognitive abilities like memory, recall, and logical

thinking. Alcohol can deplete these functions, so healthy fats are important (*6 Proven Reasons Why Your Brain Needs More Fat*, 2023).
- **Vitamins and Minerals**: Essential vitamins and minerals are important to keep things running smoothly, from B vitamins and vitamin D to minerals like iron and zinc.
- **Processed Foods, Junk Food, and Caffeine**: You should *avoid* these things. Processed foods, junk foods, and caffeine are all subtly addictive, which can undermine your recovery process while harming your physical health through unnatural preservatives and stimulating chemicals.

Ensuring your meals and snacks reflect a mix of the important nutrients, while avoiding or only consuming processed or unhealthy foods in moderation, isn't just about sticking to a diet. Keeping up with healthy eating habits means that you're giving your body the components it needs to recover from the toll alcohol has taken on it.

Superfoods for Recovery

Superfoods might sound like a modern buzzword, but they're foods packed with high levels of much-needed nutrients that can supercharge your recovery. For instance, consider the humble beetroot, which is high in betaine, a compound that helps repair liver cells damaged by alcohol abuse (Kathirvel et al., 2010). Then there's turmeric, with its active compound curcumin, which boasts powerful anti-inflammatory properties to soothe your body's aches from the inside out (Peng et al., 2021). Integrating these superfoods into your diet can help you strategically use food to support your recovery journey.

Meal Planning Tips

If you're thinking, "This sounds great, but how do I start?" then meal planning might be just the thing you need. When it comes to meal planning, it's smart to start simple. Plan your meals around a protein source, add various vegetables, incorporate a good fat source, and round it out with a complex carb. If it makes things easier, prepare your meals in bulk where you can in order to save time and stress. For instance, cook a batch of quinoa or roast a tray of mixed veggies at the start of the week. You can use these staples all week and include them in many versatile meals. It also helps if you prepare for snacking urges by keeping fruits, nuts, and yogurt handy for when hunger strikes.

When I was learning to eat healthy, I challenged myself to try a new recipe that incorporates a superfood or a new nutrient-rich ingredient each week. This built up my nutritional repertoire and kept mealtime exciting and enjoyable—a far cry from the meals I remember (or don't) from my drinking days. If you're looking to take your nutrients from zero to hero, then this challenge might be perfect for you, too.

THE ROLE OF EXERCISE IN SOBRIETY: BUILDING STRENGTH AND REDUCING STRESS

It's easy to negate the benefits of exercise. I mean, it's only a way to gain muscle or lose weight, so if you don't want to do those things, it doesn't matter ... right? Well, not quite.

Exercise is way more than that; it helps you craft a healthier, happier you. Exercise, as we've talked about, provides your brain with endorphins that make pain—mental and physical —easier to manage as you recover. The boost of endorphins and beneficial neurochemicals that you can gain from exercise is invaluable as your body and mind adjust to life without the artificial highs of alcohol.

Finding What's Right for You

But how do you find an exercise routine that doesn't feel like a chore or another daunting task on your to-do list? You can start by exploring activities that genuinely make you smile. Exercise doesn't have to be working out at the gym, but it also doesn't have to be yoga. The key is to choose an activity that you look forward to—something that feels less like a workout and more like a reward. It could be as simple as playing fetch with your dog—yes, that counts, too! The goal is to integrate this activity into your routine seamlessly and sustainably. If you love nature, hiking trails might offer the dual benefit of exercise and connecting with the outdoors. If you thrive in groups, a team sport might keep you active and expand your social circle. Remember, consistency is more achievable when you're having fun.

Setting Fitness Goals

Now, let's talk about setting fitness goals because, without them, it's easy to drift. However, these aren't going to be your run-of-the-mill New Year's resolutions that you struggle to remember by February. These goals should be realistic steppingstones that lead to genuine progress with your physical health. You can set goals that fit your exercise of choice, like walking 10,000 steps daily or attending three yoga classes weekly.

These goals should stretch you but not strain you. A goal to exercise 40 hours a week isn't going to be sustainable because it'll wear you out, and being unable to meet such a taxing goal will discourage you. In contrast, each small victory from a sustainable goal adds a brick to your foundation of self-esteem, proving to yourself that you can commit to something and see it through—which, of course, has positive implications for your recovery as well.

Exercise Is Great for the Mind

Exercise isn't just a remedy for the body; it's a tonic for the mind. The connection between physical and mental health is profound. Regular physical activity can act like a pressure valve for stress, releasing tension in a healthy, productive way (Childs & de Wit, 2014). It enhances your sleep quality, sharpens your focus, and stabilizes your mood, which can be particularly turbulent during recovery. I have never heard someone say, "I just walked around the block and I feel worse than before I did that".

Incorporating exercise into your recovery process is more than just a great way to stay fit. Keeping a look out for your body and mind through exercise also helps in creating a lifestyle where physical health is a *priority*, not an afterthought, which nurtures your mental and emotional well-being. In turn, this helps you build a body and mind equipped to handle whatever life throws your way without reverting to old patterns. This approach to exercise is a fundamental component of your new, sober life, supporting your recovery and enhancing your overall joy and satisfaction in life.

SLEEP HYGIENE: RESTORING NATURAL SLEEP PATTERNS AFTER QUITTING ALCOHOL

Ah, sleep—the elusive nightly vacation that seems to dodge you more often than not, especially after you've kicked alcohol to the curb. It can be such a challenge to get proper rest, even more so if you're used to relying on alcohol to soothe you to sleep. Sleep isn't just a luxury and a good way to relax; it's an unavoidable component of your recovery toolkit, and sleeping well is important for you to heal, inside and out. Sleep stitches up the wear and tear of daily life, both mentally and physically. Proper sleep can transform everything from your mood to your energy levels, making it a necessity.

That said, let's talk business about the sleep disturbances that often come knocking during early sobriety. It's common to find the sandman stingy with his magical sand during this time. You might find yourself tossing, turning, replaying the day, or worrying about tomorrow. Alcohol might have been your shortcut to snooze-ville, and without it, your body has to relearn how to initiate and maintain sleep naturally. Don't worry—you're not missing out by not being able to lull yourself to sleep with a drink. Alcohol-induced sleep is often restless, leaving you less refreshed than when you went to bed. Still, this readjustment period can be a real struggle, but don't fret. There are strategies to tame this beast.

Creating a sleep-conducive environment is a good starting point. Your bedroom should be like a cave—and no, I'm not playing around. Research shows that the best sleep environments should be relaxed, quiet, cool, and dark (Deshong, 2022). Because of this, it's a good idea to invest in blackout curtains to keep it dark, and maybe a white noise machine to drown out distracting noises. Keep your gadgets out of the bedroom. Yes, this means parting ways with your smartphone and binge-watching habits at bedtime. The blue light from screens can trick your brain into thinking it's party time, not sleepy time (*Does the Light from a Phone or Computer Make It Hard to Sleep?*, n.d.). Instead, spend some time cultivating a presleep ritual that tells your body it's time to wind down. This can be anything from reading a book to gentle stretches or a warm bath.

Handling insomnia proactively involves more than just setting the stage, however, because insomnia can sometimes be quite vicious. This means engaging with habits that encourage consistent sleep patterns. For example, stick to a sleep schedule—go to bed and wake up at the same time every day, even on weekends. This regularity tells your body's internal clock when it's time to go to bed and wake up, reducing the guesswork your brain has to perform. If sleep still plays hard to get, don't lie in bed wide-eyed. Get up, go to another room, and engage in a quiet, soothing activity until you feel sleepy. This prevents your mind from associating the bed with a battleground of frustration, keeping it a sleep sanctuary.

If these tips sound like they aren't going to cut it, and after you try them you find yourself staring at the ceiling night after night, it might be time to call in the cavalry—professional help. Persistent insomnia is a health hazard, dismantling everything from your cognitive functions to your emotional stability. A sleep specialist can offer insights and treatment options beyond bedtime routines, helping tackle underlying issues that might keep you awake. They can provide tailored strategies that align with your specific circumstances, ensuring your sleep strategy supports your sobriety with the precision and care you deserve.

MONITORING YOUR PROGRESS: HEALTH MILESTONES IN SOBRIETY

When you're reshaping your life without alcohol, every little win is a gold star on your chart—it matters and is worth celebrating. Setting health milestones is both a pat on your back and a clear indicator of where you've been and where you're heading. Think of these milestones as your checkpoints in a marathon. Reaching each one can give you a burst of energy and motivation to keep going, especially when the finish line seems a bit too far.

Similar to setting goals, start by setting some clear, achievable health milestones that you can use to identify your progress. You can start with something like making it through your first week alcohol-free, then stretch it out—three months, six months, a year. These milestones can also be tied to physical activity or a health goal. For instance, maybe by the three-month mark, you aim to be able to run a 5K or have successfully integrated a 10-minute meditation into your daily routine. The act of achieving these goals is just another reinforcer for your commitment to sobriety and boosts your confidence in managing your life without alcohol.

Celebrate these victories! If you acknowledge the hard work and effort you've put in, you're likely to continue making that same forward motion a habit. Treat yourself to a new workout outfit at one milestone, a professional massage at another, or a weekend retreat to mark your first sober anniversary in style. These celebrations are tangible rewards that underline your progress and inspire you to continue.

Tracking Progress: Tips and Tricks

Tracking your physical improvements can be incredibly eye-opening and encouraging. Rather than using markers like weight loss, think about how you can consider your health improvements in terms of your personal goals. You can think about your improvement in terms of achievements like:

- improved energy levels, where you feel energized for longer throughout the day
- recognition that things that previously left you out of breath no longer do
- increased mobility, flexibility, or range of motion
- meeting daily goals or following along on challenges

Please keep a record of these improvements, no matter how small they seem, so that you can look back on each and every one. They are proof of your body reclaiming its strength and vitality.

Pay attention to the importance of medical markers as well. Regular check-ups with your doctor can provide concrete data on how sobriety benefits your physical health. Improvements in liver function, blood pressure, and cholesterol levels are undeniable clinical evidence that your decision to quit alcohol is rejuvenating your body. Share your victories with your doctor and discuss them in your support groups. Sometimes, hearing a medical professional say, "You're doing great," can be the extra nudge you need to keep going. I went to the doctor every month to have my liver counts tested. Each time, my results improved, and after three months of no alcohol, they were normal again.

Mental and Emotional Improvements

Reflecting on your emotional and psychological growth is equally vital. Sobriety heals both the body and the mind, and keeping track of how your mind is improving can be awe-inspiring. For instance, you might start to notice that you're handling stress more effectively and that things that used to send you spiraling now get a calm, measured response. You may also find yourself enjoying social interactions more because you're fully present—not fogged by alcohol. Take the time to capture these reflections in a journal or through an app where you can always look back on those reflections and see how far you've come. Writing down your thoughts and feelings also helps you process them more deeply and gives you a tangible way to track your emotional evolution.

As we work to solidify your recovery, remember that taking care of your physical and mental health, as well as monitoring your progress through health milestones, is part of what helps you stay oriented on what can be a dizzying path to sobriety. Each stride forward you take toward health is worth recognizing, no matter how small. Keep these tools in hand as we progress and continue setting, reaching, and celebrating those milestones.

STEP #8

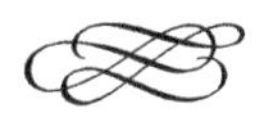

CULTIVATING MENTAL AND EMOTIONAL HEALTH

My first therapist told me that my mind is like a garden—while it can bloom with all sorts of colorful flowers, it can also harbor some pesky weeds that need to be cleared out for the excellent stuff to thrive. Stepping into sobriety, you might find that alcohol was a temporary pesticide, masking the weeds but not removing them. I used alcohol to hide anxiety, grief, and other mental health concerns, which is why learning to cultivate mental and emotional health was so important for me—and is for you, too. As you embrace a more precise, sober life, it's time to put on your gardening gloves and get to work. Step eight is about digging deep, pulling out those weeds, and nurturing your mental and emotional garden with everything it needs to flourish.

BUILDING RESILIENCE: TECHNIQUES FOR MENTAL AND EMOTIONAL STRENGTH

Resilience is the mental and emotional muscle that flexes and adapts, no matter what life decides to toss your way. It's what helps you bounce back from negative situations with a positive and proactive mindset, keeping alcohol from being your confidant or shield from dealing with the bad stuff. The inner strength of resilience lets you face a storm and leave the other side ready for a rainbow. In the context of recovery from alcohol addiction, resilience is your best friend. It supports you when you're tempted to reach for a bottle and picks you up when you feel down after a tough day. Building this resilience is a natural part of the process of maintaining long-term sobriety.

Positive Self-Talk

Positive self-talk is a powerful resilience builder. Self-talk refers to the inner monologue you have that dictates how you speak to and about yourself. Right now, it's possible that your self-talk isn't all that positive. Self-talk allows you to replace the "I can't" or "I'm not" with "I can" and "I am." When you catch yourself spiraling into negative thoughts, pause and reframe those thoughts. Think about whether the negative statements you're thinking are actually true. For example, I learned to replace "I can't handle this" with "I've handled tough situations before, and I can do it again." Simply rephrasing those thoughts and affirming the true, more realistic thoughts to myself helped reinforce my abilities and worth. Using positive self-talk to do the same for yourself can bolster your confidence and resilience.

Support Networks

Believe it or not, your support network plays an instrumental role in reinforcing your resilience. Sobriety is hard to manage on your own, even if you're pretty sure that you have things down. There might be a day when you feel the grip of alcohol stronger than ever or a day when you're not sure if you're on the right path. This is where the comfort of your support network—your friends, family, and others—can be invaluable. They can offer advice and comfort, reminding you of how far you've come already and where you have the potential to go. Maintaining a resilient mindset means leaning on those who are there for you.

Developing a Growth Mindset

Lastly, learning from setbacks through a growth mindset is an essential part of building resilience. It's easy to view mistakes or relapses as failures, but what if you saw them as valuable lessons instead? When you have a growth mindset and believe that you can develop skills and strengths through efforts, each setback teaches you something about your triggers, emotional needs, or areas where your coping strategies might need beefing up. After a setback, take some time to reflect on what led up to it. Instead of beating yourself up, take setbacks as a chance to learn and evolve on your road to recovery. Every challenge is an opportunity to strengthen your resilience.

Building resilience in recovery is a dynamic, ongoing process, and it involves cultivating a toolbox of strategies that support your mental and emotional health, nurturing a supportive network, and learning from every experience. With each step, you're moving away from your past life of addiction and toward a stronger, more resilient version of yourself. Keep flexing those resilience muscles and watch as they carry you through recovery and beyond.

THE ART OF SELF-COMPASSION: OVERCOMING GUILT AND SHAME

On the road to alcohol-free living, guilt and shame come up to bat more often than not, at least at first. These two can sneak into your thoughts constantly, whispering reminders of past missteps and poor choices. Understanding the difference between them is like distinguishing between a common cold and the flu—they're related but affect you differently and require different approaches to heal. And if you were thinking of ignoring it, leaving guilt and shame unattended is a no-go because they can fester and lead to further setbacks or relapse. So, let's chat about these two influences.

Managing Guilt and Shame

Guilt is an emotion where you feel wrong about something you've done. It's specific and tied to an action, like feeling guilty for missing an important event because you were hungover. Your conscience says, "Hey, that wasn't cool," and you feel upset because of that voice. Shame, on the other hand, goes deeper. It's about feeling wrong about who you are. A voice whispers, "You missed that event because you're a bad person." See the difference? Guilt can be a helpful nudge toward making amends or doing better next time, but shame tells you that you're not good enough to make that change.

In instances where guilt or shame are trying to wreak havoc, what you need is to treat yourself with the same kindness you'd offer a good friend if they were in your shoes. That's called self-compassion. It's a skill that involves realizing that you're human and you make mistakes, which is completely okay. Through self-compassion, you can change the internal dialogue that bounces around in your mind from one of criticism to one of understanding. Practicing self-compassion can start with mindfulness, which is just noticing your thoughts and feelings without judgment. Catch yourself when you begin to spiral into self-criticism. In these moments, pause. Take a breath. Offer yourself kindness instead, such as through a simple mantra or affirmation like, "I'm learning, and that's okay."

Being Kind to Yourself

Self-kindness is another beautiful facet of self-compassion that's related to the above. When you are kind to yourself, you're actively soothing yourself when you're in pain instead of ignoring your discomfort or punishing yourself. If it helps, think of it as treating yourself like you would a loved one who's hurting. You might tell that person to take a break when they're overwhelmed instead of pushing through until they break down or encourage them to speak to themselves gently, acknowledging their efforts and progress. This advice that you would share with your friend or loved one is the exact same advice you should share with yourself.

Letting Go of Past Mistakes

Letting go of past mistakes is an instrumental part of this process. Holding onto those mistakes is like carrying a backpack filled with stones on a hike; it slows you down and makes the journey much harder than it has to be when, really, you can just drop the backpack. Forgiveness, particularly self-forgiveness, is how you can drop that backpack once and for all. Forgiving yourself doesn't mean forgetting or excusing what happened, and it's not the same as absolving yourself from responsibility. Instead, it means accepting your past actions, learning from them, and then putting them down so you can move forward, lighter and wiser. A helpful strategy here can be writing a letter to yourself discussing the mistake, what you've learned, how you've changed, and, most importantly, offering forgiveness.

Celebrate Yourself

Celebrating yourself may sound odd at first, especially as a form of self-compassion. We're often taught to be humble and to downplay our successes. But, in recovery, celebrating your efforts and progress is a powerful affirmation of your worth. Take time to recognize your victories, no matter how small. Did you make it through a tough day without a drink? That's a win. Have you reached out for help instead of isolating? Another win. These celebrations reinforce your belief in your worth and support your journey to sobriety.

As you nurture this art of self-compassion, you'll likely notice a shift in how you view yourself and interact with the world. Self-compassion breeds a kind of peace and acceptance that can greatly impact your relationships and how you face challenges. It allows you to be your own ally, not your critic. So, next time you find yourself wrestling with guilt or shame, remember to offer yourself some compassion. After all, you're doing your best, and that's enough.

JOURNALING FOR MENTAL AWARENESS

Throughout the book so far, I've prompted you to journal a bit about different things. If you haven't noticed by now, journaling is kind of amazing. When you journal, you get to put your thoughts onto paper—or your phone or laptop, if you prefer—instead of allowing those thoughts to bounce around in your head. This gives you a structured environment in which you can explore your thoughts freely, which is definitely a positive aspect of the practice. Beyond that, when you spend some time journaling, you give yourself a log of things to look back on—you can look and see how you felt on certain days or after certain events, noticing patterns and progress alike.

When it comes to addiction, a journal can be your best friend. You can confide your deepest, darkest secrets to your journal and never have to think about the journal telling Sarah, Susie, or Bob about them. This means that you don't have to live with guilt or shame and can instead get those feelings "out there." A journal can also be a therapeutic tool that you can bring to sessions, allowing your therapist or counselor to learn more about you.

Journal Prompts for Alcohol Addiction Recovery

If you haven't started with a journal yet, you don't have to feel afraid of the process. Staring at a blank page or screen with no idea of what to write might seem terrifying, but you can use these journal prompts to give you some direction:

- Describe the moment you realized you needed to seek help for your addiction. What emotions did you feel, and what motivated you to take that step?
- Write about three things you are grateful for today. How do these things support your recovery journey?
- Identify your common triggers for drinking. How do you plan to cope with these triggers moving forward?
- Who are the key people in your support system? How have they helped you in your recovery?
- How have you changed as a person since beginning your recovery journey? Highlight both small and significant changes.
- Write a letter to yourself or someone you feel you need to forgive. Focus on the healing power of forgiveness.
- What new, healthy habits have you developed to replace drinking? How do these habits make you feel?
- What are your short-term and long-term goals for your life without alcohol? How do you plan to achieve them?
- Describe your self-care routine. How does each activity help in your recovery process?

- Write about a recent challenge you faced and how you overcame it without turning to alcohol. What did you learn from this experience?
- What are the signs that you might be slipping toward a relapse? What is your plan to prevent it?
- How are you feeling today? What emotions are you experiencing, and what might be causing them?
- Write down five positive affirmations that resonate with you. How do these affirmations help you stay strong?
- What kind of legacy do you want to leave behind? How do you want your recovery journey to inspire others?
- Imagine your life five years from now as a sober individual. Describe it in detail. What are you doing, how do you feel, and who is in your life?

You can use these prompts more than once to give yourself deeper insight into the same situation, or you can even make up prompts of your very own. Don't be afraid to journal as much as you need. You can even journal creatively by recording videos, painting, or dancing to express your emotions—it's less about the medium and more about self-expression.

MORE SELF-REGULATION TIPS FOR THE JOURNEY

Rounding off your toolkit a bit, let's touch on some additional self-regulation tips that can help as you recover.

Deep Breathing Strategies

Breathing might not seem like much. I mean, you breathe all the time. How much can breathing help? A lot, actually! Deep breathing strategies are known to regulate your nervous system, which can lessen your stress and help you feel more in control (*Stress Management: Breathing Exercises for Relaxation,* n.d.). Some of my favorite breathing strategies for emotional regulation include:

Strategy	Steps
Diaphragmatic Breathing	1. Sit or lie down in a comfortable position—be that your bed, couch, or even the floor. 2. Place one hand on your chest and the other on your stomach. 3. Inhale deeply through your nose, allowing your stomach to rise while keeping your chest relatively still. Allow your hand to measure the breaths and feel the sensation of your belly inflating. 4. Exhale slowly through your mouth, feeling your stomach fall. 5. Repeat for 5-10 minutes, focusing on the rise and fall of your abdomen as the hand on your chest stays still. You can switch hands every few minutes if you'd like.
4-7-8 Breathing	1. Inhale gently through your nose for a count of 4. 2. Hold your breath for a count of 7. 3. Exhale completely through your mouth for a count of 8. 4. Repeat the cycle four to eight times.
Box Breathing	1. Inhale through your nose for a count of 4. 2. Hold your breath for a count of 4. 3. Exhale through your mouth for a count of 4. 4. Hold your breath again for a count of 4. 5. Repeat the cycle for 3-5 minutes.

Alternate Nostril Breathing	1. Sit comfortably with your spine straight. 2. Close your right nostril with your right thumb. 3. Inhale deeply through your left nostril. 4. Close your left nostril with your ring finger, release your right nostril, and exhale through your right nostril. 5. Inhale deeply through your right nostril. 6. Close your right nostril with your right thumb, release your left nostril, and exhale through your left nostril. 7. Continue this pattern for 5-10 minutes.

Pursed Lip Breathing	1. Inhale slowly through your nose for a count of 2. 2. Purse your lips as if you are going to whistle. 3. Exhale gently through your pursed lips for a count of 4. 4. Repeat for several minutes, focusing on the slow, controlled exhale.

In wrapping up this exploration of cultivating improved mental and emotional health, remember that each step you take toward an improved mindset and each skill you gain is part of what will cement your recovery in stone. While they won't assure that you never face a challenge—because nothing can truly do that—they are a safeguard that can keep your recovery clear from the hands of addiction. Next up, we'll take a look at how strengthening personal relationships is a vital part of your journey.

STEP #9

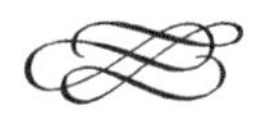

REBUILDING AND STRENGTHENING PERSONAL RELATIONSHIPS

We've talked about it a lot by now—your relationships are going to change as you maintain sobriety. For me, it went like this. I was at a family after years of not attending, and I was suddenly the center of attention —not for the usual antics of days gone by, but because I was now the non-drinker in the room. People were all walking on eggshells around me, both because they were afraid I would explode into a relapse or snap at any moment and because they didn't quite know what to say. The relationships there were certainly strained, and it wasn't the first time that happened to me.

When you become sober, every social gathering can feel like your debut as the new, sober you. These affairs can range from reconvening with old friends to meeting new ones, with each interaction necessitating careful navigation. As the ninth step, we're unpacking these interactions and giving you a roadmap to social success.

COMMUNICATING YOUR SOBRIETY: SHARING YOUR JOURNEY WITH LOVED ONES

The people who matter most to you are probably the same people you will want to talk to about your journey, including your reasons for and your progress. However, it can be really difficult to have those conversations. It starts with honesty.

Honest Conversations

Honest conversations are the first step in rebuilding and strengthening relationships. These are the conversations where your voice and your heart are present, letting those around you know about your experiences in a candid way. When you open up about your sobriety, you can definitely say, "I don't drink anymore." But for some friends and family, you might want to be a bit more specific in sharing a piece of your journey. For this, you need vulnerability.

To have honest conversations about your journey, start with the people closest to you, those who've been there through thick and thin. In reality, you can tell anyone you want about your journey, but starting with those closest to you is going to be an easier process. As far as you are comfortable, talk to them about the what and the why of your recovery. You can tell them about the moments that led to your decision, the challenges, and the triumphs.

It's completely normal for others to ask you questions when you do share. You can, of course, open up, but if you aren't comfortable with sharing certain information, just let them know. It's as easy as saying, "I'm not ready to share that part of my story, but I would love to talk to you about that someday."

Educating Family and Friends

While your family and friends love you, they might have a bit of a hard time getting the complete picture of what overcoming alcohol addiction involves. They might not understand what it involves or why it's a big deal. It can be hurtful to be met with questions like, "What's the big deal? You can just stop whenever you want." This is where a little education goes a long way.

Because you're the main source of connection that your loved ones have to recovery, you can be the one to help them understand. Remember how I said personal stories can help people understand by making them more relatable? Your family and friends will get it way faster if they have a personal connection—you. If they have questions, break down what addiction and recovery mean. Maybe bring resources to a family dinner or share articles or videos that resonate with you to help back you up. This can make interactions with family members go from tolerance to informed support. This educational moment can turn misunderstandings into meaningful dialogues, replacing myths with facts and assumptions with understanding.

Receiving Support

Asking for support through recovery might feel like asking someone to help you move—it's a big ask. But unlike lugging a sofa up three flights of stairs, support in your sobriety journey can be as simple as having someone to call when you're feeling low or finding someone who'll swap out pub crawls for coffee catchups. Let your loved ones know what type of support you need, and be specific. Is it calling you every Friday night or joining you for a morning walk? Remember, people often want to help but don't always know how. Guiding them not only eases your path but also deepens your mutual connection.

Celebrating Small Victories Together

Every step forward in your sobriety journey deserves a high-five, whether it's your first week sober or your first year. Share these milestones with your loved ones instead of just celebrating them alone. Maybe throw a sober birthday party or have a small family dinner where you can express your gratitude for their support. Celebrating these victories together not only marks your progress but also reinforces the shared journey. It turns your victories into collective celebrations and makes your loved ones an active part of your recovery. Plus, these shared moments of joy can strengthen your bonds like nothing else.

Communicating about your sobriety means that you are continuously inviting your loved ones into your world, helping them see the world of addiction recovery through your lens. It's a process, a sometimes messy, sometimes beautiful process where words and emotions are shared, misunderstood, and then understood through honesty and transparency. While these communications might not always go how you want or expect, each word shared is a step toward understanding. Each moment of education is a bridge being built. You're not alone, and when you're rebuilding relationships, you create a network of support that surrounds you with strength, understanding, and love.

HEALING BROKEN BONDS: MAKING AMENDS AND REBUILDING TRUST

When making amends, think of it as less as uttering a quick "sorry" and more like repairing a home chipped away at by the elements over time. You can't slap some plaster on it and call it a day; sincerity must be fused into your apologies, patching up past hurts with genuine acknowledgment of your actions and reinforcing the foundation of your relationships with a commitment to change. Making amends goes beyond the surface—it addresses the underlying issues your actions may have caused. This requires a thoughtful approach and an understanding of the difference between a simple apology and a heartfelt amendment.

Let's break it down. An apology often comes in the moment, a quick response to an immediate mistake. "I'm sorry I was late" is an apology that acknowledges a mistake but doesn't necessarily correct the action or make up for it. Making amends, however, involves acknowledging the ripple effects of your actions. Making amends means not only taking responsibility for being late but also recognizing how your delay may have made the other person feel undervalued or disrupted their plans. Saying, "I'm sorry," and exploring how to prevent this issue in the future, perhaps by managing your time better or communicating earlier if you're running behind, is the start of the process of making amends. This process isn't solely a means of clearing your conscience but rather a way to rebuild trust through actions that speak louder than words.

As an active addict, there were probably many times when you hurt someone or broke their trust because of your relationship with alcohol. Even if you didn't mean to do it, addiction hurts those around you, and it's your responsibility to rebuild the trust lost by every missed event, hangover-induced lack of responsibility, and party crashed by excessive drinking. Rebuilding trust is something that requires consistency in your actions and reliability in your commitments. Someone who no longer trusts you doesn't have to start trusting you again immediately, but you can still make efforts to improve trust and give that person a reason to trust you again. For example, if you say you're going to call, call. If you promise to be there, show up. These actions might seem minor, but they add up. Over time, these small, consistent actions accumulate, restoring faith in your reliability and integrity.

During this process, you need to know how to handle rejection and disappointment. Not everyone will be ready to accept your attempts to make amends, and that's okay. People heal on their own timelines, just like how you're healing from addiction, and sometimes, despite your best efforts, they might not be ready to mend the bond, or they may never be. This can be tough to digest, but in these moments, respect their feelings and give them space. Focus on what you can control—your actions and responses. Also, be sure to use this as an opportunity to practice patience and understanding, recognizing that their inability to forgive does not reflect their worth or sincerity in making amends.

Lastly, healing broken bonds requires forgiveness, particularly self-forgiveness. You have to accept that while you cannot change the past, you can learn from it and move forward. Forgiving yourself releases a heavy weight you've been carrying and empowers you to understand that making mistakes doesn't make you unworthy of love or redemption. Extend this forgiveness to others as well. People make mistakes and might have acted in ways that hurt you during addiction, but it's important to be willing to forgive them, too. Just as you hope others will forgive you, offer them the same grace. This mutual exchange of forgiveness can be immensely healing, creating a future for yourself where past wounds no longer define the relationships you have with others.

In navigating the complex world of making amends and rebuilding trust, be sure to remain patient. It's, of course, desirable to have relationships mended overnight just by sobering up, but not everyone works that way. If someone repeatedly made choices that hurt you, you would struggle to trust them, too. Over time, that trust can come back with continued effort. Just remember that that effort has to continue even after the bond has been repaired for it to stay that way. Continue spreading knowledge, compassion, and forgiveness, and the people who matter will be bonded with you more strongly than ever.

SETTING HEALTHY BOUNDARIES: PROTECTING YOUR SOBRIETY IN RELATIONSHIPS

When you rekindle your relationships, it's easy to try and make everyone happy by bending your boundaries. Someone might try to convince you that it's just one drink and that it won't hurt, and you might feel compelled to give in to make them happy or avoid a conflict. Situations like these only highlight just how important it is to have healthy boundaries, especially in social situations where drinking is involved. It's not necessarily *fun* to set these boundaries, but they are a necessity to safeguard the life you're rebuilding.

Identifying when and where you need these boundaries is the first step to setting healthy boundaries that maintain your progress. Knowing your limits is important, and you can identify your limits by asking yourself questions such as:

- What situations make you feel uncomfortable or at risk?
- Who in your circle tends to make recovery more challenging?
- What social changes would make you feel more comfortable in terms of your recovery?

Recognizing these situations—or people—that contribute to making your recovery uncertain can help you anticipate and prepare rather than react and regret. This is what being proactive looks like. For example, if you know that a particular cousin always brings up triggering topics, you might need to limit your time around them or have a plan to change the conversation to proactively maintain your social safety.

When communicating our boundaries, many of us feel a tug-of-war between guilt and assertion. No matter how you feel about it, you absolutely have to work on laying your boundaries out clearly and kindly. In order to do so, choose a calm, neutral time to talk, not in the heat of the moment. Use "I" statements to express your needs without blame. For example, say, "I need to leave by 9 p.m. to keep to my routine," instead of, "You don't respect my limits." This way, it's about your needs, not their actions. Be as specific as you can—vagueness breeds misunderstandings. Also, people who genuinely support your sobriety will respect these boundaries, even if they don't fully understand them.

Now, respecting your own boundaries can sometimes be trickier than setting them. It's easy to bend your rules, especially if you feel pressured or want to avoid conflict. But every time you uphold your boundaries, you affirm to yourself that your recovery matters. Conversely, disregarding your own boundaries can set you back and even trigger a relapse, which is why it's important to stand by your boundaries even if in-the-moment pressure is strong. For instance, if you've committed to leaving a party early, stick to it, even if you're having a good time. It's not just about that one night; it's a symbol of maintaining the integrity of your boundaries and your trust in yourself.

Another thing to think about when it comes to setting boundaries as you improve your social relationships is dealing with boundary violations. People might forget your boundaries, and some people might even violate your boundaries to test the waters and see if you're serious. When this happens, address it immediately. Let's say a friend forgets and brings wine to your dinner party. Take them aside, remind them of your boundary, and ask them to respect it next time. If violations persist, you may need to consider more serious actions like distancing yourself from that relationship. It's tough, yes, but protecting your sobriety has to come first. It's better to have two friends who respect you and your boundaries than twenty who don't.

SUPPORTING OTHERS: HOW TO BE THERE FOR FRIENDS AND FAMILY FACING ADDICTION

When it comes to addiction, the person with the addiction isn't the only one who feels it. Their friends, family, and anyone in their immediate circle will also feel the effects of it, and this time, I'm not talking about you. As someone with an addiction to alcohol, it's not unlikely that other people you know also face addiction—be it to alcohol or something else. In these situations, it can be so tempting to try and extend a hand and just fix it for them, but that's not how it works. That person doesn't need you to fix it for them; they need you to be a supporter for them. If you know someone with an addiction and walk to be there for them, I'll help explain to you how you can show up for them.

Empathy and Understanding

Supporting someone else who is facing an addiction starts with empathy and understanding. As someone who has dealt with addiction yourself, you probably already have some idea of what they're going through. Or, if you're reading this book as someone without an addiction and looking for ways to help, you might have no idea. Either way, empathy and understanding are important, and it doesn't take that first-hand experience to get there.

Addiction is a complex beast, often clouded by misconceptions and stigma. To support someone, you have to be willing to see beyond the addiction and recognize the human struggle beneath, which can be a challenge when addiction is so pervasive in their life. This means listening to their experiences, fears, and hopes without judgment, even if you yourself have had similar experiences. Sometimes, the most powerful thing you can do is offer a safe space for them to express themselves. This can be as simple as saying, "I'm here if you want to talk," and then just sitting with them, whether they open up or in silence. Empathy is about connection, not correction. While you can't walk the path for them, you can walk beside them, offering your presence as a source of comfort and strength.

Avoiding Enabling

Something else to be mindful of is the balance of supporting a loved one through addiction without enabling them. We talked about this earlier. Enabling often starts with good intentions. You might think taking over their responsibilities will ease their stress and lead to a reduction in their addiction. However, doing this can prevent them from facing the natural consequences of their actions, which are often crucial motivators for seeking help or committing to change in the first place.

Instead of doing this, focus on supporting your loved one in ways that empower them. For instance, instead of lending money, which they might spend on substances, offer to help them budget or find financial counseling. If they're really struggling, rather than handing over money, you can offer to take them grocery shopping instead, encouraging independence while offering support in a less enabling way. It's also good to encourage activities that contribute to their well-being, like attending a support group meeting or cooking a healthy meal. Remember, genuine support encourages growth and independence; it doesn't foster dependency.

Encourage Professional Help

Encouraging professional help can sometimes feel like convincing a cat to take a bath—there's resistance. However, recommending that someone with an addiction seek professional health is something that you have to approach gently and respectfully. It always helps to start by expressing genuine concern for their well-being based on observations, not judgments. "I've noticed you've been seeming really down lately" is more constructive than "You've got a problem." From there, you can suggest that they consider talking to someone who can provide professional guidance, emphasizing that it's a sign of strength, not weakness, to seek help. Offer to help them research therapists or rehab facilities or to be there for moral support when they make that first call. Sometimes, knowing they don't have to do it alone can make all the difference.

Look Out for Yourself, Too

Lastly, don't forget about yourself in this equation. Supporting someone through addiction recovery is no small feat, and it's easy to get so caught up in their health that you sideline your own. Trying to support someone without looking like yourself is the same as trying to pour water from an empty cup—eventually, you run dry. Maintain your mental and emotional well-being by setting aside time for activities that replenish your spirit, and remember to keep your boundaries clear. It's okay to say no if supporting them is compromising your health. After all, you can offer the most help at your best.

Closing out this chapter, it's important to remember that while rebuilding and strengthening relationships can be complicated, it's possible and completely worthwhile. From communicating your sobriety decisions and making amends to supporting others and setting boundaries, each stride you make fosters relationships that support your new sober life. Finally, for our last chapter together, we'll explore how engaging with a broader community can enhance your recovery journey, offering new perspectives and fresh support networks. Keep your heart open and your boundaries firm, and your journey will continue to unfold with each step you take.

STEP #10

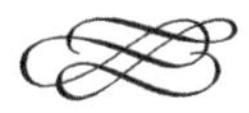

CREATING AND LEVERAGING A SUPPORTIVE COMMUNITY

I never thought I would be able to walk into a room where everyone just ... understood. They understood that we all faced unique struggles, and many of the people faced struggles similar to mine. It was something I never thought I would have again—a supportive community. But through hard work and dedication, I forged a community of my very own. Like-minded people on their paths to sobriety surround me now, and it's so inspiring to have so many positive people around me.

As step ten in this journey, you are going to find your tribe and safety net, where shared experiences and wisdom collide to create something beautiful. Don't worry; we're almost to the end of the book, and you've done an amazing job at taking the initiative to heal. With this last step, you'll have everything you need to embark on a journey to sobriety that is powerfully and uniquely your own.

FINDING YOUR TRIBE: CONNECTING WITH SOBER COMMUNITIES AND GROUPS

The right people for us don't fall from the sky, as convenient as that would be. Instead, you have to know where to look to find people just like you who are willing to be a part of your journey, and a great place to connect is within the welcoming walls of sober communities.

Benefits of Sober Communities

The magic of connecting with sober communities lies in the shared journey. No one understands the struggles of alcohol addiction better than someone who has experienced it first-hand, and the benefits of connecting to others who share a similar path are astounding.

First off, the aspect of feeling understood deeply and genuinely can be incredibly healing. Each shared story reminds you that you're not alone in this and that your struggles and victories are part of a larger movement toward recovery. These communities also offer a treasure trove of resources—from coping strategies and insights into navigating social situations to recommendations for therapists and sober-friendly activities. You don't have to feel like each coping strategy is hiding because communities like these are more than willing to share. And let's not overlook the accountability factor—people in such communities are often willing to share in keeping you accountable for your own sobriety, which is motivational beyond words.

How to Find Local and Online Groups

So, where do you find these mythical bands of sober warriors? It's best if you start by looking at your own local community. Check out community centers, libraries, or even local cafes for bulletin boards with meeting information. Hospitals and clinics often have details on support groups, too. And don't forget your trusty friend, the Internet. A quick search for "sober communities" or "recovery groups" along with your location can bring up a ton of options. Websites like Meetup can be great for finding local groups or events centered around sobriety. For those who prefer tapping into support from the comfort of their homes, online forums and social media groups offer a platform to connect with global communities, providing support at the click of a button. I belong to several private groups on Facebook. The encouragement there is spectacular, offering support from day one of sobriety to years later, through relapses, and all the challenges that alcoholics face during recovery.

All of this is to say that finding a community that's right for you doesn't have to be hard. Whether you vibe more with face-to-face interactions or prefer the comfort of a computer, there is something out there for you and plenty of ways to find that "something."

Engaging With Sober Activities and Events

Diving into sober activities can add another layer of joy and connection to your life by offering fulfilling activities and connections. Many communities organize sober hikes, book clubs, dance classes, or art workshops. These activities and events can help fill the leisure time you might have previously spent drinking and strengthen your connections with others in the community, building friendships based on shared, sober fun. This, in turn, helps you redefine enjoyment and relaxation in ways that support your lifestyle.

Creating Your Supportive Community

Perhaps you've searched far and wide and still can't find a group that clicks—or you're just bursting with ideas for sober activities. Why not start your own group? Creating a community allows you to tailor activities and discussions to fit your vision of support and recovery, and you never know —your vision just might be perfect for tons of other people, too. To gain a community, try inviting a few folks from your existing social circles who are also on a sobriety journey, or reach out to people looking for support. Choose activities that encourage interaction and camaraderie, like starting a sober book club or a morning coffee meet-up.

ONLINE RESOURCES AND SUPPORT: NAVIGATING THE DIGITAL SOBRIETY LANDSCAPE

Welcome to the digital age, where support, guidance, and community are just a click away! The internet is an incredible place where you can find people, tools, information, and help at the click of a button, no matter the time or place. The internet itself is kind of like a support group in this way, and you can certainly take advantage of the resources and support that you find online as a part of your journey. Whether you are looking for shared stories to inspire you, seeking advice at 2 a.m., or tracking your sober days, the digital world has your back.

Leveraging Online Platforms

First, you can explore the vast online platforms that cater to people who are navigating sobriety. These communities offer spaces where you can connect to people just like you, usually with the intention of sharing your experiences or advice with others. Websites tailored to addiction offer social networking and professional resources, thus creating a space to connect with peers, share your experiences, and access recovery tools all in one spot. Then, educational sites like The Recovery Village provide valuable information about addiction and recovery and offer direct paths to professional help. You can also find supportive people in groups tailored to addiction on ordinary social media platforms like Facebook and Reddit, which takes some of the stress out of trying to find a you-specific group.

Digital Support Groups

Now, let's talk about digital support groups. Digital support groups are often structured as forums, meeting rooms, and chatrooms where you can reach out to people who are going through the exact same struggles. These virtual rooms are where stories are shared, encouragement is doled out in generous portions, and advice flows from one person to the next. Platforms like "In The Rooms" and "DailyStrength" host numerous support groups for various aspects of recovery, including specific groups for alcohol addiction. These forums allow you to dive into discussions, ask questions, or read others' experiences. Such an opportunity can provide you with a sense of community that can be lifesaving on tough days.

Apps for Sobriety

There's nothing more convenient than having the tools you need for sobriety right in your back pocket. By this, I mean the little device you own called a smartphone, which is home to dozens of apps that contribute to sobriety support. Apps like "I Am Sober" or "Nomo" are fantastic for tracking your sobriety milestones, logging daily emotions, and connecting with a community that cheers on each day you add to your sober streak. These apps, and many similar apps, usually include features like daily motivational quotes, progress trackers, and the ability to share your achievements with friends or within the app community. Imagine getting a badge for every week, month, or year you stay sober—a digital pat on the back that can boost your morale and motivate you. That's exactly what these apps can do for you.

Maintaining Privacy and Safety Online

While the digital world is rich with resources, navigating it safely can sometimes be challenging. The internet is a public space, after all, and protecting your privacy is always something to keep in mind first and foremost. When engaging in online forums or support groups, consider using a pseudonym or at least avoid sharing highly personal information like your full name or exact location. It's shocking just how much someone can find out about you by knowing that you're Abby from Chicago, and even if their cyber-tactics can't force a bottle into your hands, they can still make your life a challenge, especially if you're trying to keep your addiction on the down-low for the moment.

Also, be cautious about the links you click and the personal data you share. Links can often be disguised as something innocuous, and some people are unnecessarily cruel, even to those already navigating a tough time. Never click on links or hyperlinks, and if you're really curious, try to find the link on Google instead of clicking it directly. Most reputable sites and apps will have robust privacy policies as well—read them. Never give any websites you don't trust your financial information either. If you're ever in doubt, a good rule of thumb is to share only what you would be comfortable having a stranger know. After all, safeguarding your personal information should be as much a priority as maintaining your sobriety.

Navigating the digital landscape of sobriety resources offers a world of information, support, and community at your fingertips, all for the low cost of your internet bill. Immersive platforms, supportive online groups, handy apps, and all the information you can possibly desire can be found on the internet, which can significantly bolster your recovery efforts. As you continue to explore and utilize these digital tools, remember that they are supplements to your overall recovery strategy—valuable, accessible, and empowering resources that can help you build and sustain a sober, fulfilling life.

VOLUNTEERING AND GIVING BACK: HOW HELPING OTHERS CAN SUPPORT YOUR RECOVERY

Crafting this book has been my contribution to the broader recovery community. To me, this is a gesture of solidarity and support to those embarking on their path to sobriety. I wrote this book with the hope that my experiences, transformed into written words, will light the way for others, offering both solace and practical guidance. Alongside this project, maintaining a journal has become a therapeutic practice for me, enabling me to navigate my emotions and reflections and, in turn, foster a deeper understanding of my recovery journey. These endeavors have been acts of giving and played an important role in my ongoing healing process, illustrating the profound interconnectedness of helping oneself while reaching out to help others.

I'm telling you this because I want you to know that it doesn't take much to give back. You can write a book about your experiences and share it with the world, create art that represents your journey, or even volunteer to help others as a means of giving back. I especially recommend volunteering as an easy yet meaningful way of fulfilling yourself while helping others out. When you step out of your own life and immediate responsibilities to help someone else, you're doing a good thing that helps you *feel* good, all while creating a cycle of positivity that uplifts others and boomerangs right back at you. In this way, volunteering becomes a cycle of positivity for you and anyone you extend your kindness to.

The Value of Service

So, why does volunteering feel so darn good? When you help others, your brain creates the very same dopamine and endorphins we talked about earlier when we discussed the benefits of exercise. It's nature's little reward system, cheering you on for making a positive impact. Volunteering is able to do this because when we help others, we recognize the difference that we can make in the world and understand just how much that impact can change someone's life. It's something you *should* feel good about!

More than just the biological buzz, volunteering also reinforces your sense of purpose. It's easy to become trapped in uncertainties and future recovery possibilities, and it's also easy to let the negative parts of life in general get you down. Making a tangible difference in someone else's life is a powerful reminder that you have the ability to make valuable contributions to the world around you and that the world isn't all doom and gloom, even if it feels that way from time to time. Your actions matter, which can be a powerful antidote to feelings of inadequacy or self-doubt that might try to sneak into your sober life.

Finding Volunteer Opportunities

Opportunities to volunteer are all around you; many places are constantly looking for volunteers to support the community in one way or another. Personally, I recommend that you start with what you love. Passion fuels persistence, so pick causes that ignite a fire in your heart. For example, if you're an animal lover, local shelters are often on the lookout for volunteers. If you're a bookworm, how about helping at the library or reading to kids at the community center? For those who've found strength through their recovery process, consider roles that allow you to support others battling addiction. Many rehabilitation centers and community recovery organizations welcome individuals willing to share their time and experiences. To find these opportunities, tap into local community boards, visit nonprofit websites, or even a simple Google search can lead you to volunteer opportunities in your area.

The Impact of Helping Others

To you, a day of volunteering might have felt like a day of making a difference, but to the person you helped, it might be way more than that. Have you ever really taken a moment to notice how a single act of kindness can turn someone's day around? That simple day being transformed can show them how kind the world can be, uplifting them and carrying them through not just a day but a week or longer.

Now, imagine that impact multiplied; that's what volunteering can do. When you volunteer, it creates more of an impact because there are more people volunteering, which means more lives are touched by your willingness to give back. It also fosters a sense of connection and community, which can help keep your recovery process in forward motion. Feeling part of something larger can significantly dilute feelings of isolation or loneliness that are common in those of us managing recovery.

Psychologically, helping others can boost your self-esteem and provide a fresh perspective on the world around you.

When you take the time to volunteer and help others, be they human lives or animal lives, that time you spend serves as a reminder that everyone has struggles and that you are not alone in facing challenges. Plus, the gratitude you receive—spoken or implied—when you volunteer is often a heart-warming affirmation that you are making a difference, which can be incredibly uplifting and affirming.

Setting Healthy Boundaries in Service

While volunteering is undeniably beneficial, you also have to approach it with a strategy that supports your recovery. Setting boundaries for volunteering matters because when you're making a difference, it can be easy to overexert yourself or overcommit, and then it can be a challenge to bow out when you need to. Avoiding this means having a plan for what you can handle and what fits your needs as you serve others.

Before you dig into a long-term volunteering project, decide how many hours you can commit each week without feeling overwhelmed. Make sure that you're also choosing volunteer roles that don't trigger stress or jeopardize your sobriety. For instance, if large groups drain your energy, look for opportunities that involve working in smaller teams or even solo tasks. It's also okay to say no or to step back if your volunteer work starts to feel like a burden rather than a joy. Your well-being is the priority, and the right volunteer fit should feel like a natural extension of your recovery, not something that makes your recovery more challenging.

Helping others is just as much about them as it is for you. In recovery, volunteering and giving back in any way means that you're giving yourself the gift of joy and fulfillment. Each act of service supports those in need while contributing growth, connection, and self-worth to the overall dynamic of your sober life.

STAYING INSPIRED: KEEPING SOBRIETY FRESH AND ENGAGING

Believe it or not, sobriety can get a bit boring sometimes. When you're working toward the same thing for so long, it can be a bit tiring to continue working toward the same goal in the same way. If you're feeling like this at any point in your process, you need to change things up with a sprinkle of daily inspiration, a commitment to growth, and the courage to face new challenges.

Finding Inspiration in Recovery

As you know by now, recovery isn't just a process where you stop drinking and call yourself recovered. Instead, recovery is a continuous learning process where you find new ways to love and enjoy a life that is separate from the addiction that once gripped you. There are so many places where you can find inspiration to learn and grow:

- **Books**: Books can be an amazing source of inspiration. Fiction or non-fiction, reading about the stories of others is a way that you can find knowledge and inspirational wisdom that propel you forward in the recovery process. For instance, *This Naked Mind* by Annie Grace shifts perceptions about alcohol and can change how you view sobriety.

- **Podcasts**: Podcasts speak to you, literally, while telling you about the experiences of others and offering insight into how you can frame your recovery based on the latest knowledge, research, and understanding of sobriety. Podcasts like *Recovery Elevator* or *The Bubble Hour* provide insightful discussions and share personal stories of recovery that might mirror your own or open new windows of understanding.
- **Interviews**: Celebrity interviews or interviews from recovered individuals are like a window into your future and a mirror of your past. You can use interviews to understand how other people's paths have unfolded and what yours might look like down the road. This helps you change or develop your journey according to your long-term goals.
- **Social Media**: Social media is often a place of negativity, but with the right care and mindful consumption, the accounts and posts of people who have recovered are incredible sources of inspiration for your continued journey.
- **Real People You Know**: There doesn't have to be this elusive layer of separation between you and those from whom you derive inspiration. Real people you know can be inspirations, too!

Renewing Your Commitment

As days turn into weeks and weeks into months, you might find your initial zeal for sobriety waning a bit. It's natural for this to happen. This is the perfect time to renew your commitment to sobriety, which can be super helpful for "refreshing" your recovery. I mean, think about how some people renew their vows. It's not because they lost their love for one another, but rather to refresh their commitment to one another. In order to do the same thing for your recovery, reflect on why you chose this path and celebrate how far you've come. Maybe renewing your commitment means revisiting your goals or setting new ones, like improving your physical health or learning a new skill that supports your sober lifestyle. It might also mean re-engaging with your support groups or a therapist if you've stepped back a bit. Think about what would make you feel renewed in your commitment and work with that as your guiding force.

Continuous Growth and Learning

Adopting a mindset of continuous growth and learning keeps you on track and improves your ability to grow as you learn more and more about yourself through recovery. Every day offers a new lesson, and a fresh opportunity to expand your understanding of yourself and refine your approach to challenges. It would be best if you considered engaging in workshops, seminars, or classes focusing on personal development that allow you to keep learning, even after you consider yourself "recovered." Topics like stress management, emotional intelligence, or even creative writing can offer you tools to handle the emotional and psychological demands of sobriety. These learning opportunities keep your mind engaged and your spirit enthusiastic about each day's growth. And always remember, growth often comes dressed up as challenges, so embrace them as chances to learn rather than obstacles.

Embracing New Challenges

Speaking of challenges, think of challenges as a new adventure just waiting to be explored. This might sound overly optimistic, but beating yourself up has never gotten you very far. Instead, embrace a sense of growth and use challenges as a chance to move you forward along your path. This might look like taking on a new role in your job, trying out a new sport, or even volunteering for an important cause. It can also look like turning a failure into your biggest rebound. Things that push you out of your comfort zone are where growth happens. In these moments, when you're a bit uncertain and testing your limits, you often discover just how much you're capable of.

ADVOCATING FOR SOBRIETY: BECOMING A VOICE FOR POSITIVE CHANGE

When you think about advocacy, it's easy to think of someone with a megaphone at the front of a bustling rally, but let's dial it back a bit—advocacy comes in many shapes and sizes and is way more accessible than you might think. Advocacy, especially regarding sobriety, can start with something as simple as sharing your story. Turning your personal journey into a powerful tool that challenges societal views and lights a path for others who might still be struggling in silence is advocacy. Each time you share your story, you're also chipping away at the massive wall of stigma that surrounds addiction. I recently told one of my coworkers that I don't drink anymore because I am an alcoholic. She looked very surprised, so I said, "There is nothing wrong with being an alcoholic!". She agreed and told me I was right and she shared that she had quit drinking because her liver counts where abnormal. Everyone knows someone who is effected by alcohol and sharing you successes helps others. You're showing the world that recovery isn't only possible but worth celebrating—and celebrating *loudly.*

Sharing Your Story

Sharing your story doesn't mean you have to stand on a stage with all eyes on you—unless that's your thing, of course. It can be something as intimate as a blog post, a podcast, or even a chat over coffee with someone curious about your sobriety. The key here is authenticity. Being honest and raw about the ups and downs, the setbacks and successes of your recovery is way more important than spreading your story to as many people as possible. Your story, shared honestly and candidly, shows that sobriety isn't a linear path paved with constant joy; it's a real human experience filled with challenges and triumphs. Each time you open up, you shed light on your journey and illuminate a path that could guide someone else out of their darkness.

Do not hesitate to share your journey. My experiences with opening up, even to those I barely knew, have been entirely positive. Each conversation about my journey, theirs, or that of a loved one was met with encouragement and gratitude. Being transparent has helped my personal recovery and inspired others too. On one occasion, my dental hygienist inquired if I would consider speaking at a conference like her son-in-law, a possibility I might explore later on—probably sometime after you close the cover of this book. The opportunities to make a difference are boundless when you approach them with openness and honesty.

Involvement in Policy and Advocacy

If you're feeling particularly inspired to take a difference, why not take your advocacy a bit further? Engaging in policy and advocacy efforts directly leads you to the changes you want to see in society. This might come in the form of lobbying for better funding for addiction recovery programs or pushing for laws that support recovery integration, like job protections for those undergoing treatment. Getting involved might sound daunting, but you can start by reaching out to local representatives or join existing organizations that fight for policy changes in addiction recovery. Recovery is often met with a lot of roadblocks, and your help in shaping better social and political attitudes won't go unnoticed by those hoping to recover.

As you step into the role of an advocate, remember that your voice has power. No matter how you choose to use that voice, your push for meaningful change can ripple far beyond what you might see. So, grab that metaphorical megaphone and let your advocacy speak volumes, both for your journey and for countless others who might just be waiting for a sign to start their path to recovery.

THE ROLE OF MENTORSHIP IN SOBRIETY: BEING A GUIDE FOR OTHERS

Mentorship is another incredible way that you can contribute to creating and leveraging a supportive community—especially if your aim is to be a part of that community for others. Becoming a mentor in the sobriety community means you're sharing your time, your experiences, strengths, and hopes, which can significantly impact someone else's life. But what does it take to be a good mentor? It takes empathy, reliability, and a solid understanding of your sobriety.

For starters, mentoring others must always come from a place of empathy and warmth. Remember those early days, the struggles, and the victories? Holding those memories close allows you to connect deeply with those you mentor. It's so important for those just beginning their journey to have a safe and understanding space for them to navigate their challenges, and your mentorship creates that space. Listening, really listening, and responding with kindness and wisdom is part of the role as well. Then there's reliability, something non-negotiable if you hope to create a relationship of trust. What I mean is that being a mentor requires you to be consistent and show up mentally and emotionally for meetings or check-ins.

At the same time, mentorship isn't just about guiding—it's also about setting boundaries. As a mentor, strong boundaries protect both your well-being and the integrity of the mentor-mentee relationship. Those boundaries are what tell you how deeply to involve yourself in a mentee's challenges without overstepping or taking on their burdens as your own. For example, while it's important to be accessible when your mentee needs you, you might want to set specific times for calls or meetings, thus making sure that you have time to recharge and attend to your own needs. This helps maintain a healthy balance, allowing you to be there for them without compromising your sobriety or emotional health, or accidentally lapsing into a relationship of enabling.

For mentees, the benefits of having a mentor are clear: Guidance, support, and an inspiring example of successful sobriety. But for you, the mentor, the rewards are equally as enriching. Mentoring others can reinforce your recovery journey by reminding yourself of the strategies that worked for you and why you chose sobriety. It's a way to reaffirm your commitment and reflect on your growth. Moreover, mentoring enhances your sense of purpose and can be incredibly fulfilling.

If you choose to go the route of being a mentor, you should be sure to schedule in time when you can reflect on the experience. Reflecting on the mentorship experience encourages you to consider how far you've come and how your journey can motivate and help others. Taking the time to really reflect also gives a chance to see the impact of your efforts and watch someone else grow because of your guidance. Through reflection, you can take pride in your mentorship and improve your ability to help others as a mentor.

CONTINUOUS LEARNING: EDUCATING YOURSELF AND STAYING INFORMED ON ADDICTION AND RECOVERY

The process of recovery doesn't have a finish line. Whether you're still working on your own recovery or have moved to supporting others alongside yourself, educating yourself and staying informed is necessary. We know quite a bit about addiction and recovery on many levels—scientific and psychological just to name a few—but that doesn't mean that we know everything. The realm of addiction and recovery is broad and ever-evolving and staying informed empowers you with knowledge and the tools to handle your sobriety with finesse.

The Importance of Ongoing Education

Alright, I hear you asking, "Why should I stay educated when I already know about addiction first-hand?" The fact of the matter is that you're never going to know everything. Continuous learning provides guidance and helps you understand the intricacies of addiction, the psychological underpinnings, the latest in recovery methods, and even relapse prevention strategies. This knowledge means that you can support yourself and others in your community using research-backed information. While older, more familiar methods can seem comforting, the world is always evolving and so must our approach to addiction. When you engage in ongoing education, you help yourself, better understand your behaviors and triggers and equip yourself with strategies to deal with challenging days.

Resources for Learning

There are many places where you can take a look at resources that are up-to-date and constantly evolving when it comes to addiction research. While books can't change as readily as webpages, and therefore are harder to update, books like *Alcohol Explained* by William Porter and *The Unexpected Joy of Being Sober* by Catherine Gray can help you understand the biological factors behind addiction. They transform complex scientific concepts into relatable, understandable nuggets of wisdom that can keep you up to speed on some of the trickier concepts to understand.

Also, websites like SAMHSA (Substance Abuse and Mental Health Services Administration) offer resources, access to community programs, and up-to-date research that are constantly being updated to ensure that people like you and I are never in the dark about the latest findings on addiction and recovery. For a more interactive learning experience, you can take a look (or listen, rather) to podcasts such as *Recovery Happy Hour* and *Sober Cast*—these options provide real-life insights and stories of recovery that you can listen to from anywhere, turning your commute or jog into a mini-classroom.

Attending Workshops and Conferences

Ongoing learning can be even further improved by attending workshops or conferences, either about addiction or alcohol directly or about topics that feel related—like relationships, substance abuse, and similar. At these events, conversations invite you to improve your knowledge base and gain a deeper understanding of the nuances you might not be able to pick up on your own. After all, we as individuals can't really understand the whole of addiction solely from our personal experiences. Listening to experts and engaging with a community as committed to recovery as you are is inspiring, educational, and informative when it comes to keeping up with the latest details that can help you support yourself or those around you.

Sharing Knowledge With Others

You don't have to keep all of that insight you gain through continuous learning to yourself. Think about the last time you learned something exciting and how you couldn't wait to tell someone about it. Sharing what you know can be helpful for yourself and for others, creating an excellent chance for conversation and to be helpful all in one go. Sharing this knowledge can be as simple as discussing a new coping strategy you read about over coffee with a friend or as formal as leading a session in your local support group. Sharing knowledge creates a culture of learning and growth within your community where people are unafraid to ask questions and feel that their path is brighter and less scary.

EMBRACING A NEW IDENTITY: THE TRANSFORMATIVE POWER OF SOBRIETY

Stepping into sobriety gives you the unique opportunity to embrace a whole new version of yourself. People constantly change, and everyone will go through many identities throughout their lifetime for one reason or another. Like shedding old skin that no longer fits, finding your new identity after recovery really allows you to be the person you are now instead of the person that addiction made you out to be. Finding a new identity means getting in touch with who you are, all through a newfound lens of recovery.

Redefining Yourself Beyond Addiction

Let's start with the big makeover: Redefining who you are without the shadow of alcohol looming over you. Initially, this might feel awkward to try and do since alcohol and drinking might have been a big part of your life for quite a while. You can begin the process of exploring who you are outside of addiction by exploring interests that alcohol always prevented you from trying.

If you're not sure where to start, try thinking about a trait you've always wanted to have, but never had the chance to develop. For example, if you always really wanted to be creative, take a look at some creative hobbies that you can use as an outlet. On the other hand, if you always wanted to be more sporty but alcohol kept you too sedated, think about a sport you might want to try. Recovery gives you a chance to almost start over in a sense, and you can take that opportunity and run with it, wherever it may lead you.

The Role of Sobriety in Shaping Your Identity

As you delve into this new sober lifestyle, you'll notice it's a process involving more than avoiding a beer at dinner; it's a lens that magnifies what's important to you. Sobriety has a sneaky way of reshaping your priorities and values, and it's definitely not a bad type of sneaky. Sobering up and maintaining that lifestyle means that your mind is now clear to see what matters to you the most. You might gravitate toward genuinely supportive relationships or develop a newfound appreciation for honesty with yourself and others. You might find that your favorite activities were just an effect of alcohol, and now you realize that you're freer to be who you truly are. As sobriety helps you align your daily life with your actual values, you'll feel more congruent and more authentic.

Navigating Changes in Self-Perception

Adjusting the mirrors of self-perception does have its challenges, I won't lie. Initially, you might struggle with a skewed self-image, where you feel like your failures have more weight than your accomplishments. Here's where you need to tune into a different frequency. Don't let those negative thoughts take hold and tell you that you're less than incredible, and instead, start affirming your worth daily. Remind yourself of your strengths, both in and outside of recovery. Keeping a gratitude journal where you make note of things you're grateful for about yourself and your recovery is an amazing way to start this practice, as is the creation of positive affirmations that you can repeat to yourself for inspiration.

Celebrating the New You

Imagine throwing a party where the guest of honor is the new, sober you—what a bash that would be! Celebrating this new identity that you create through recovery is part of the process of making sure that recovery isn't something you'll lapse out of. Making the time to celebrate who you're becoming and the progress you've made is a necessary step that reinforces the positive changes and highlights your commitment to maintain them. Celebrate your sober anniversaries, but don't leave out the minor victories either — like the first time you say no to a drink at a party, the first month you fill with new hobbies or the first conflict you navigate with clarity and grace.

As you embrace your new, sober identity, remember that sobriety doesn't mean that you have to deny yourself what you love—it's actually the opposite. Being sober means rediscovering the things you love and the passions that you have in a more authentic, sustainable way. Under this new personality, you can trade the temporary highs of alcohol for the lasting satisfaction of hard-earned progress. Each step you take in redefining yourself, from exploring new interests to reshaping your values and celebrating your growth, is a step toward a life where you are thriving because of your sobriety.

Creating a community for yourself and leveraging that community to your benefit comes in a lot of shapes and sizes. Your friends and family are part of your community, but so are the people in your support groups, online, and who you mentor. Your new personality, who you truly are, is also a part of this group and shouldn't go unnoticed either. Learning, growing, and always keeping a look out for yourself and your community is going to make the world go 'round when it comes to harnessing a recovery that feels both fulfilling and complete.

A Chance to Spread Hope

There's a new chapter ahead of you, one that's far brighter than the past you've been dealing with. As you set forward into its pages, take a moment to share inspiration with someone else who needs this transformation.

Simply by sharing your honest opinion of this book, you'll inspire other people struggling with alcohol addiction to take those essential first steps – and you'll show them exactly where they can find all the guidance they need to get there.

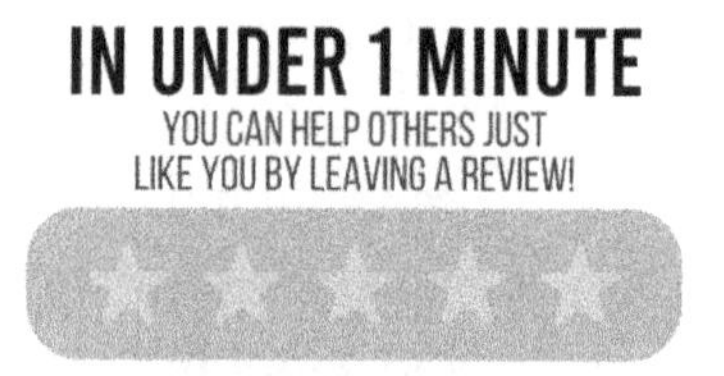

Thank you so much for your support. I wish you a bright and healthy future.

Scan the QR code below

Or Put this link into your browser

https://www.amazon.com/review/review-your-purchases/?asin=
B0D9CCTL7Z

CONCLUSION

Well, here we are at the end of our shared journey—a path that's taken us from the dark valleys of alcohol addiction to the hopeful peaks of sobriety. Reflecting on this path, it's clear that the road to recovery is both challenging and amazing, and that's all a part of the process. Together, we've explored the emotional whirlwinds, the physical hurdles, and the psychological battles that come with breaking free from alcohol's tight grip. Remember those stories I shared with you and the big themes we worked through together? Each was a step—a lesson on this trek from struggle to strength.

Understanding addiction was our starting point, recognizing it not as a sign of weakness but as a complex condition that can hijack the brain, body, and soul. We debunked those pesky myths about alcoholism and learned to view it as a medical issue deserving of empathy and informed care rather than judgment.

But we didn't stop at understanding; we moved to action—those 10 simple yet impactful steps I laid out for you. From sparking that initial motivation and laying a solid foundation for sobriety to making meaningful lifestyle adjustments based on the foundation of understanding and strengthening your support circles—each step was designed to guide you toward a healthier, sober life.

Improved health, deeper relationships, and a sense of community are just a few of the advantages waiting for you at the end of your addiction. A life where clarity replaces confusion, where each morning is greeted not with regret but with anticipation is no longer something you have to yearn for. It's a very achievable reality available to you, right here and now.

As you close the cover of this book, keep in mind that the journey doesn't end here. Sobriety is an ongoing process of growth and learning. Keep feeding your curiosity, seeking support, and exploring new passions that fill your life with joy and purpose. The road to recovery is long and perpetually paved with opportunities to learn more about yourself and the world around you.

Oh, and don't forget to keep your support system close as you walk through each step of this guide. Whether it's family, friends, or fellow travelers on the road to recovery, surround yourself with people who understand, care, and can provide a shoulder or a cheer when needed. You're not in this alone, and the strength of your network can be the strength you draw from on the more challenging days.

Now, please take a deep breath. It's time to embrace this sober life you've been preparing for. Use the steps we've discussed, lean on your support network, and start walking forward—one day at a time. With each step, remember that you're moving toward a life of freedom, health, and abundant possibilities.

As we close off this journey together, I just wanted to let you know that you are capable. You are stronger than you think, and you are worthy of the incredible life on the other side of addiction.

Thank you for walking this path with me. Here's to your health, happiness, and new, alcohol-free life. Cheers (with sparkling water in hand, of course) to new beginnings and your continued success on this journey!

REFERENCES

5 common fears in recovery and how to overcome them. (2024). ArmsAcres. https://www.armsacres.com/blog/fears-in-recovery

6 proven reasons why your brain needs more fat. (2023, August 23). Grey Matters of Carmel. https://greymattersofcarmel.com/brain-health-fat-diet/

Alcohol and Drug Foundation. (2021, October 4). *Understanding dual diagnosis.* ADF. https://adf.org.au/insights/understanding-dual-diagnosis/

Alcoholic liver disease Information. (n.d.). Mount Sinai Health System. https://www.mountsinai.org/health-library/diseases-conditions/alcoholic-liver-disease

Alcoholism statistics you need to know. (2018, January 23). Talbott Recovery. https://talbottcampus.com/resources/alcoholism-statistics/

American Addiction Centers Editorial Staff. (2016, September 29). *Total alcohol abstinence vs moderation: Which one wins in the end?* DrugAbuse.com. https://drugabuse.com/blog/total-alcohol-abstinence-vs-moderation-which-one-wins-in-the-end/

Baum, E. (2022, December 16). *How to celebrate sobriety milestones.* 7 Summit Pathways. https://7summitpathways.com/blog/how-to-celebrate-sobriety-milestones/

Bharadwaj, B., & Kattimani, S. (2013). Clinical management of alcohol withdrawal: A systematic review. *Industrial Psychiatry Journal, 22*(2), 100. https://doi.org/10.4103/0972-6748.132914

Bridges of Hope. (2023, May 20). *What to eat when going through withdrawal and detox.* Bridges of Hope Rehab Treatment Center. https://bhoperehab.com/what-to-eat-when-going-through-withdrawal/

Carbohydrates. (n.d.). Heart. https://www.heart.org/en/healthy-living/healthy-eating/eat-smart/nutrition-basics/carbohydrates

Casali, M. (2021, December 17). *Acute withdrawal vs. protracted withdrawal.* Turnbridge. https://www.turnbridge.com/news-events/latest-articles/acute-withdrawal-vs-protracted-withdrawal/

Childs, E., & de Wit, H. (2014). Regular exercise is associated with emotional resilience to acute stress in healthy adults. *Frontiers in Physiology, 5*(161). https://doi.org/10.3389/fphys.2014.00161

Cleveland Clinic. (2022a, March 14). *Neurotransmitters: What they are, functions & types*. Cleveland Clinic; Cleveland Clinic. https://my.clevelandclinic.org/health/articles/22513-neurotransmitters

Cleveland Clinic. (2022b, April 25). *Gamma-Aminobutyric acid (GABA)*. Cleveland Clinic. https://my.clevelandclinic.org/health/articles/22857-gamma-aminobutyric-acid-gaba

Clinic, A. R. (2023, November 6). *Overcoming alcohol addiction: 4 inspiring stories of triumph and transformation*. Aquila Recovery Clinic. https://www.aquilarecovery.com/blog/overcoming-alcohol-addiction-4-inspiring-stories-of-triumph-and-transformation/

Cohen, M. (2022). *Signs you're enabling a loved one's addiction*. WebMD. https://www.webmd.com/mental-health/addiction/features/addiction-enabling-a-loved-one

Deshong, A. (2022, December 13). *Sleep environment: Temperature, humidity, light, & noise*. Sleep Doctor. https://sleepdoctor.com/sleep-environment/

Does the light from a phone or computer make it hard to sleep? (n.d.). KidsHealth. https://kidshealth.org/en/teens/blue-light.html

Eddie, D., Bergman, B. G., Hoffman, L. A., & Kelly, J. F. (2022). Abstinence versus moderation recovery pathways following resolution of a substance use problem: Prevalence, predictors, and relationship to psychosocial well-being in a U.S. national sample. *Alcoholism: Clinical and Experimental Research, 46*(2). https://doi.org/10.1111/acer.14765

Foundation, G. (2018, June 7). *Voice of Recovery: Craig*. Gateway Foundation. https://www.gatewayfoundation.org/addiction-blog/alcohol-success-story/

Get to know carbs. (n.d.). ADA. https://diabetes.org/food-nutrition/understanding-carbs/get-to-know-carbs

Hjalmarsdottir, F. (2018, October 15). *17 science-based benefits of omega-3 fatty acids*. Healthline; Healthline Media. https://www.healthline.com/nutrition/17-health-benefits-of-omega-3

Kathirvel, E., Morgan, K., Nandgiri, G., Sandoval, B. C., Caudill, M. A., Bottiglieri, T., French, S. W., & Morgan, T. R. (2010). Betaine improves nonalcoholic fatty liver and associated hepatic insulin resistance: a potential mechanism for hepatoprotection by betaine. *American Journal of Physiology-Gastrointestinal and Liver Physiology, 299*(5), G1068–G1077. https://doi.org/10.1152/ajpgi.00249.2010

Mary Jo DiLonardo. (2010, October 6). *What Is alcohol withdrawal?* WebMD. https://www.webmd.com/mental-health/addiction/alcohol-withdrawal-symptoms-treatments

McInally, J. (2023, December 21). *What are alcohol withdrawals? Symptoms, treatment & timeline*. Home Alcohol Detox Treatment London, UK. https://www.detoxtoday.co.uk/how-to-deal-with-alcohol-withdrawals/

MINDFUL STAFF. (2020, July 8). *What is mindfulness?* Mindful. https://www.mindful.org/what-is-mindfulness/

Murray, K. (2020, May 6). *Types of therapy for alcoholism*. Alcohol Rehab Guide. https://www.alcoholrehabguide.org/treatment/types-therapy-alcoholism/

Peng, Y., Ao, M., Dong, B., Jiang, Y., Yu, L., Chen, Z., Hu, C., & Xu, R. (2021). Anti-Inflammatory Effects of Curcumin in the Inflammatory Diseases: Status, Limitations and Countermeasures. *Drug Design, Development, and Therapy, 15*, 4503–4525. https://doi.org/10.2147/DDDT.S327378

Pinelands Recovery Center Staff. (2022, January 10). *Benefits of drinking water in addiction recovery*. Pinelands Recovery Center of Medford. https://www.pinelandsrecovery.com/benefits-of-drinking-water-in-addiction-recovery

Post-acute-withdrawal syndrome (PAWS): An in-depth guide. (2018). American Addiction Centers. https://americanaddictioncenters.org/withdrawal-timelines-treatments/post-acute-withdrawal-syndrome

Rios, T. T. H. O. L. (2023). *The power of tea: 100 health and wellness benefits*. The Tea House on Los Rios. https://theteahouseonlosrios.com/blogs/news/the-power-of-tea-100-health-and-wellness-benefits

Sarkar, D., Jung, M. K., & Wang, H. J. (2015). Alcohol and the immune system. *Alcohol Research : Current Reviews, 37*(2), 153–155. https://www.ncbi.nlm.nih.gov/pmc/articles/PMC4590612/

Sissons, C. (2018, July 10). *8 foods that boost serotonin naturally*. Www.medicalnewstoday.com. https://www.medicalnewstoday.com/articles/322416

Stonebraker, C. (2023, September 29). *What is pink cloud syndrome in recovery? Meaning, and what to expect*. The Insight Program. https://theinsightprogram.com/blog/pink-cloud-syndrome-meaning-recovery

Stress management: Breathing exercises for relaxation. (n.d.). Myhealth. https://myhealth.alberta.ca/Health/Pages/conditions.aspx?hwid=uz2255

Wang, X., Yu, Z., Zhou, S., Shen, S., & Chen, W. (2022). The Effect of a Compound Protein on Wound Healing and Nutritional Status. *Evidence-Based Complementary and Alternative Medicine, 2022*. https://doi.org/10.1155/2022/4231516

Wendt, T. (2022, September 1). *Hippocampus: What to know*. WebMD. https://www.webmd.com/brain/hippocampus-what-to-know

Wiggins, R. (2023, May 5). *The harmful effects of alcoholism on families.* Primrose Lodge. https://www.primroselodge.com/blog/relationships/the-effects-of-alcoholism-on-families/

"101 Inspiring Recovery Quotes About Addiction." Landmark Recovery. Last modified August 23, 2023. https://landmarkrecovery.com/addiction-recovery-quotes/.

Printed in the USA
CPSIA information can be obtained
at www.ICGtesting.com
LVHW091325270924
792207LV00008B/735